BEYOND
BIGGER
LEANER
STRONGER

THE ADVANCED GUIDE TO BUILDING MUSCLE, STAYING LEAN, AND GETTING STRONG

Michael Matthews

oculus

Cover Designed by Damon Za

Typesetting by Kiersten Lief

Edited by Kristin Walinski

Published by: Oculus Publishers, Inc.

www.oculuspublishers.com

Visit the author's website: www.muscleforlife.com

CONTENTS

MY STORY:
HOW I TRANSFORMED MY BODY, AND
HOW YOU CAN TOO

My mission is to empower people to take control of their health and fitness by following a healthy, enjoyable lifestyle that not only gives them the body they've always wanted but also enables them to live a long, vital, disease-free life.

I'M MIKE, AND I BELIEVE THAT every person can achieve the body of his or her dreams. I work hard to give everyone that chance by providing workable, proven advice grounded in science, not a desire to sell phony magazines, workout products, or supplements.

Through my books, I've been able to help tens of thousands of people lose weight, build muscle, and get healthy. My goal is to turn that number into hundreds of thousands and ultimately millions.

I've been training for more than a decade now and have tried just about every type of workout program, diet regimen, and supplement you can imagine. Like most guys, I had no clue what I was doing when I started out. I turned to magazines for help, which had me spending a couple of hours in the gym every day and wasting hundreds of dollars on worthless supplements each month, only to make mediocre (at best) gains.

This went on for years, and I jumped from workout program to workout program. I tried all kinds of splits and routines, exercises, rep ranges, and rep timing schemes, and while I made some gains (it's impossible not to if you just keep at it), I eventually hit the dreaded plateau.

My weight remained stuck for over a year, I wasn't getting stronger, and I had no idea what to do with my nutrition beyond eating clean and making sure I was getting a lot of protein. I turned to various trainers for guidance, but they had me do more of the same. I liked working out too much to quit, but I wasn't happy with my body, and I didn't know what I was doing wrong.

Here are a couple of pictures of me after almost 6 years of lifting regularly:

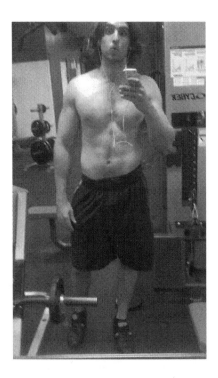

Not very impressive. Something had to change.

TIME TO GET SMART

I finally decided that it was time to get educated—to throw the magazines away and learn the physiology of muscle growth and fat loss and what it takes to build a big, lean, and strong body.

So I got serious about doing real research. I searched out the work of top strength and competition coaches, talked to scores of natural bodybuilders, and read hundreds of scientific papers, and a very clear picture emerged.

The real science of getting into incredible shape is very, very simple—much simpler than the health and fitness advice and supplement industries want us to believe. It flies in the face of almost all the crap that we hear on TV, read in magazines, and see in the gym.

Here's a small sampling of what most people will never know about getting into the best shape of their lives:

- Lifting light weights for high reps is basically a waste of time. If your routine doesn't revolve around heavy lifting, you're doing it wrong.

- Getting lean, and even super lean, does NOT require hours upon hours of grueling cardio or crash dieting that leaves you starving and miserable every day.

- If you know what you're doing, you can gain 20 to 30 pounds of lean mass (yes, muscle) in your first year of training, regardless of your genetics.

- Pretty much every machine in the gym should be avoided, and most exercises are horribly ineffective. This brings me to the next point...

- The idea that you have to constantly change your workout routine or your body will adapt and plateau is a lie. I change my routine once every 2 to 4 months and consistently get stronger month after month.

- You don't have to exercise for more than 1 hour per day, 5 days per week to be in peak physical condition. I personally lift weights Monday through Friday for about 45 minutes and do 3 or 4 cardio sessions per week, with each session running about 30 minutes. And I do the cardio mainly because I enjoy it.

There are many, many more lessons I've learned, but what it all boils down to is building a muscular, lean, and healthy body doesn't require your life to revolve around it. You can fit it into almost any schedule or lifestyle.

As a result of what I learned, I completely changed the way I trained and ate. And my body responded in ways I couldn't believe.

My strength skyrocketed. My muscles grew faster than I could ever remember. My energy levels went through the roof.

That was just over 4 years ago, and here's how my body has changed since:

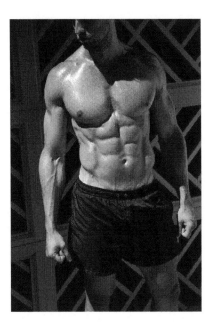

Quite a difference.

THE BIRTH OF MY CAREER

I took "hardgainers" and put 30 pounds on them in a year. I took people who were absolutely baffled as to why they couldn't lose weight and stripped 30 pounds of fat off them and helped them build noticeable muscle at the same time. I took people in their 50s who believed their hormones were too bottomed out to accomplish anything with their bodies and helped them turn back the clock 20 years in terms of body fat percentage and muscle definition.

After doing this over and over for years, my "clients" (I never asked for money—I just had them come train with me) started urging me to write a book. I dismissed the idea at first, but it began to grow on me.

"What if I had such a book when I had started training?" I thought. I would've saved an untold amount of money, time, and frustration, and I would've achieved my ideal physique years ago. I enjoyed helping people with what I had learned, and if I wrote books and they became popular, what if I could help thousands or even hundreds of thousands of people? That got me excited.

So I started by publishing *Bigger Leaner Stronger* in early 2012, unsure of what to expect. Sales were slow at first, but within a month or two, I began receiving e-mails from readers with high praise. I was floored. I immediately started on my next book and outlined several more.

I've now published seven books and sold more than 200,000 copies, and I get scores of e-mails and social media messages every day from readers who are blown away by the results they're seeing. They're just as shocked as I was years ago about how simple it is to build lean, healthy muscle and lose as much fat as you want without ever feeling starved or miserable.

It is motivating to see the impact I'm having on people's lives, and I'm incredibly inspired by the dedication of my readers and followers. You guys and gals rock.

WHERE TO NOW?

My true love is researching and writing, so I'll always be working on another book, my blog, and whatever else my writing adventures bring my way.

My big, evil master plan has three major targets:

1. **Help a million people get fit and healthy.** "Help a million people" just has a sexy ring to it, don't you think? It's a big goal, but I think I can do it. And it goes beyond just helping people look good—I want to make a dent in alarmingly negative trends we're seeing in disease and mortality.

2. **Lead the fight against broscience and BS.** Unfortunately, this industry is full of idiots, liars, and hucksters who prey on

people's fears and insecurities, and I want to do something about it. In fact, I'd like to become known as the go-to guy for practical, easy-to-understand advice grounded in real science and results.

3. **Help reform the sport supplement industry.** The dishonest pill and powder pushers are the people I despise the most in this industry. The scams are numerous: using fancy-sounding, but worthless ingredients; cutting products with junk fillers like maltodextrin and even stuff like flour and sawdust (yes, I'm not kidding); using bogus science and ridiculous marketing claims to convince people to buy; underdosing the important ingredients dramatically to save money (and using a proprietary blend to hide it); sponsoring steroid-fueled athletes to pretend supplements are the secret to their gains; and more.

I hope you enjoy this book, and I'm positive that if you apply what you're about to learn, you too can dramatically transform your physique without hating your "diet" or beating yourself to death in the gym every day.

So, are you ready? Great. Let's get to it.

THE PROMISE

If you're an experienced weightlifter but still haven't been able to achieve and maintain a muscular, shredded physique…aren't quite sure what to do next with your body…or feel like you've fallen into a rut or lost the excitement you once felt for training, then you want to read this book.

WHAT IF YOU COULD MAKE SIMPLE, but powerful, changes to how you train and eat and not only "make gains" again but get downright ecstatic about the results you see in the gym and in the mirror?

What if I showed you how to systematically pinpoint and address the weak points in your physique that, when fixed, dramatically improve your overall look?

What if I told you that even as an advanced weightlifter, you can make fantastic gains without spending more than an hour in the gym 3 to 5 days per week and without crushing yourself with drop sets, supersets, giant sets, and other similar nonsense? What if I told you this "overkill" approach actually guarantees you'll never see good progress again?

What if I showed you how to get shredded (5 to 7% body fat) without frying your muscles, metabolism, or sanity? And what if I showed you how to then maintain that super-lean physique for as long as you'd like … while staying strong … with ease?

Imagine if you knew exactly what it takes to get into such good shape that everyone will swear you're on steroids and would never believe that you're doing it without living in the gym, living off boiled chicken and steamed broccoli, or yelling at yourself for having that extra bite of dessert.

Imagine hitting the gym every day knowing that you're going to leave a little closer to your goals and that you'll never tumble into the fitness purgatory of being forever stuck at kind of big, kind of lean, and kind of strong.

And imagine never growing bored with your training or losing interest, even after 2, 4, or even 10 years. Imagine hitting the gym every day just as pumped to train as you were in your dreamy days of newbie gains.

Well, the reality is you can have all of these things and more, and it doesn't require taking out a second mortgage to hire expensive trainers, following complex dietary and training routines that drive you neurotic, clearing the shelves of GNC, or buying enough drugs to kill an elephant. It doesn't require becoming a hermit or neurotic, and it doesn't mean you'll have to risk your health or longevity.

What does it require, though?

I think you know the answer: the right know-how, above-average discipline and a strong work ethic, and a lot of consistency and patience.

These are powerful virtues to develop in ourselves. They can enrich our lives in incredible ways, the least of which is building a great physique.

This book will show you how to do all these things, no matter your age or circumstances. You can become a paragon of health and fitness—an inspiration to friends, family, and even strangers—and remain one for the rest of your life.

That's ultimately what I want for you.

I want you to look in the mirror every day for the rest of your life and beam with pride, knowing that your body is completely under your control and that you can engineer it exactly as you desire.

So, then, turn the page, and let's begin this journey together.

INTRODUCTION:
BIGGER LEANER STRONGER VS. BEYOND BIGGER LEANER STRONGER

IF YOU'VE READ *BIGGER LEANER STRONGER* (*BLS*), you might be wondering how this book differs from it and how it should be used. Should you follow the advice in *BLS* or this book? Or a bit of both? Those are good questions, so let's take a moment to address them.

This book assumes you've read *BLS*, so if you haven't and aren't already familiar with the training and dietary principles discussed in it, you're probably going to wind up confused in certain parts of this book.

We have a lot of new stuff to cover, so I wanted to avoid repeating myself as much as possible.

Think of this book as a true sequel to *BLS*—you can jump in here and enjoy yourself, but certain things aren't going to click without reading that book first.

That said, here's how I intend *BLS* to be used with this book:

1. Read *BLS* first and this book second. By the end of both of these books, you will know more about fitness than 99% of forum warriors, gymbros, and self-styled gurus.

2. If you're new to weightlifting, start with the *BLS* program, not the program in this book.

3. Use the *BLS* program for your first 1 to 2 years. In this time, you will be able to gain 20 to 40 pounds of muscle and dramatically increase your strength. Once you've reached that point, you're ready for the *Beyond Bigger Leaner Stronger* program.

4. If you're not new to weightlifting but have never trained in the way I teach in *BLS*, you too should start with that program.

5. Make the switch to the program in this book once you've reached the strength milestones given in a later chapter on the *Beyond Bigger Leaner Stronger* program.

If you're an experienced weightlifter who is no stranger to heavy, compound weightlifting, and you've met or surpassed the strength milestones given later, then you're in a perfect place to begin the *Beyond Bigger Leaner Stronger* program.

On the dietary side of things, as you'll see, the advice in this book builds directly upon the principles taught in *BLS*, and you can use them even if you're not following the training program in this book.

You can't go wrong sticking to the simple dietary rules given in *BLS*, but you may want to incorporate some of the more advanced strategies of this book.

Now, you may also be wondering why this book and a new program even exist. Is *BLS* not so great after all? Did I just need an excuse to publish another book?

While I do have a wife with expensive tastes and little boy who is quickly growing our grocery bills, I have other reasons for writing this book and for evolving the *BLS* program.

The details on why your training method changes are in a later chapter, but know that this book and the *Beyond Bigger Leaner Stronger* program are not replacements for *BLS*.

The primary purpose for this book and its program is to help you smoothly move through the toughest phase for most guys in their quest to get fit: the point when the newbie gains are long gone, where progress is slow even when you're doing everything right, and where the little things related to training and diet make all the difference.

The reality is you could stick with just *BLS* indefinitely and do great, but you'll do even better with this book under your belt as well.

So, with all that out of the way, let's get to the fun stuff, starting with the inner game of fitness, especially as it applies to us veterans of the gym game.

Specifically, I'd like to talk about how the fitness lifestyle can positively impact other areas of our lives, and why having a strong, muscular, healthy physique is much more valuable than just being able to move heavy things and look pretty.

1

WHY WORKING OUT MAKES YOU BETTER AT LIFE

FEW PEOPLE ARGUE THE MANY HEALTH benefits of regular exercise.

We all know it wards off all kinds of disease, and scientists have shown it's a great way to fight depression, improve intelligence, and protect against the cognitive decline associated with aging.

Many people don't realize that the benefits of exercise go far beyond physiological and psychological improvements, however. Achieving your fitness goals can fundamentally change you as a person. It can help you overcome your fears and weaknesses and teach you a lot about how to succeed in all areas of your life.

I believe that if you can create the body of your dreams, you have what it takes to create the life of your dreams as well.

Sounds like a stretch? Well, let me explain.

In this chapter, I want to present to you four vital life lessons I believe working out teaches us and how they affect our ability to not only build great physiques but also great lives.

THE POWER OF HABIT

When you woke up today, what did you do first, and in what order? Did you go straight to the shower? Did you check your e-mail first, or Facebook and then e-mail?

When did you brush your teeth in your routine? Which shoe did you tie first—the right or left? What did you say to your family before leaving?

What route did you drive to work? What did you do once you got to your desk? Did you go straight to your e-mail, or did you chat with a colleague first?

And what about lunch? Did you have leftovers or a salad? Or maybe a burger?

What did you do once you got home? Go for a bike ride? Pour a drink and have some dinner?

I could go on and on with these questions, but here's my point:

We truly are creatures of habit, and we all have deeply ingrained daily patterns of behavior.

In fact, according to a 2006 study conducted by researchers at Duke University, more than 40% of the daily actions people perform aren't actual decisions: they are habits.[1]

In many cases, these habits are useful. They save us mental energy. We don't need to decide each day how to put toothpaste on our toothbrush or how to go about washing our bodies.

But other habits are much more complex, can emerge without our permission, and can be quite troublesome.

For example, studies have shown that families who eat fast food regularly didn't originally intend to eat as much as they do. The monthly habit eventually became a weekly one, which eventually became a twice-per-week occurrence, until finally they're eating junk food every day.

We can fall into this trap in any area of our lives.

Thirty minutes of TV per day can become 60, and then 100, and so forth. Skipping exercise once per week leads to skipping twice per week, which eventually leads to quitting. One drink per week can, for some, easily multiply in size, frequency, or both.

The ramifications of such negative habits can be deceiving.

There are the immediate and obvious effects: you fall behind your peers in your work and are passed over for the promotion, you gain weight and feel lethargic, your health deteriorates, and so forth.

Then there's the insidious: you lose faith in your ability to put your mind to something and see it through; you avoid challenges and opportunities for fear of failure; you criticize yourself, eroding your self-esteem; you become depressed; and so on.

Habits cut both ways, though.

Forty-five minutes of exercise several days per week, if you do it over a sustained period, can transform your body. Thirty minutes of reading per day, over time, can turn you into an expert in just about anything. An hour or two of more work per day than your peers helps you produce dramatically more than them.

Much clichéd advice about achieving success focuses on the dreaming the right dreams and wishing the right wishes.

This is all well and good, but thinking dim thoughts does not make things happen. Our dreams may influence what we're capable of, but our habits will ultimately determine what kind of lives we live.

Anyone can be energized by a tantalizing vision, but very few people can stick to the daily grind long enough to get there. Fifteen seconds of fantasy can take 15 years of habitual action to fully realize.

"We are what we repeatedly do," Aristotle wrote. "Greatness then, is not an act, but a habit."

Show me a great achiever in any field or activity, and I'll show you a master of *habit*—someone who mechanically repeated the same, positive actions countless thousands of times until finally he had produced something extraordinary, whether it is a skill, fortune, invention, or even a meaningful relationship with another person.

Controlling our habits can be quite hard, though. Some routines and actions are so ingrained that we find ourselves slaves to them, unable to do anything but mindlessly comply.

Well, this leads me to one of the great unsung benefits of staying fit: it teaches us habit mastery. That is, it teaches us how to control our habits—how to break bad habits and protect good ones.

You see, you don't overcome bad habits with voodoo rituals, exorcisms, or self-denial. You beat them by simply creating new behavior patterns that overpower and override them.

Instead of watching that hour of TV every night to unwind, you let off steam with an hour of weightlifting. The enjoyment normally provided by the 3 PM cookie snack is replaced by an equally enjoyable apple with peanut butter. You trade the short-lived pleasure of junk food for the longer-lasting pleasure of improved health and overall well-being that comes with eating cleanly.

You've probably heard that it takes somewhere between 21 to 30 days to form a new habit. This rule of thumb originated with Dr. Maxwell Maltz's seminal 1960s book Psycho-Cybernetics, but actual scientific research has demonstrated it can take quite a bit longer—about 66 days on average.[2]

Interestingly enough, once you establish a new pattern, it quickly begins to feel just as automatic as the old one, no matter how different it is. Whatever we repeatedly do is what we want to continue doing, whether it's eating ice cream in front of the TV or hitting the treadmill for some late-night cardio.

In this way, achieving your fitness goals becomes easy. You just keep doing what feels right, and you make slow and steady progress. Over time, these small improvements add up to something extraordinary, even if the whole process feels natural, comfortable, and even effortless.

By doing this, you not only show yourself that you can change your behavior patterns—that you are in control—but you also come to realize how powerful your routine is. And it begins to mold other areas of your life. You become different from other people.

Many people underestimate the time and effort it takes to make things happen. They don't give much thought to the long-term habits all meaningful endeavors require. They just set off haphazardly, and they don't last long in their journeys.

As you build your habit mastery through exercise and diet, however, you begin to look at all goals differently.

You realize that new undertakings require new habits and that often old habits have to go to make room. And you know that the first month or two of a new habit is always the toughest but that it becomes more and more automatic and familiar as time goes on.

You aren't afraid of the idea that something will take 1, 2, or even 3 years of regular work to see through. You've learned patience—to appreciate the actions of today, no matter how small they might seem, for their contributions to the bigger picture.

Achieving a high level of habit mastery will give you a *huge* advantage in other areas of your life. People will talk about your superhuman work ethic and follow-through. They will marvel at the sheer amount of *stuff* you can get done.

Little will they know, however, that you don't possess any mysterious superpowers. You've just used fitness to develop a skill that many people don't have and don't understand.

TOUGHNESS AND THE WILLINGNESS TO EXERT EFFORT

Sometimes I wonder how much of our current population would survive a thousand years ago—you know, when you had to chase, fight, and kill to survive. When grueling, physical hardship was a price we paid to remain at top of the food chain.

The social veneer of modern technology and luxuries has made us soft. The basic necessities of survival are a few mouse clicks away. The problems of modern living are laughable: where are we going to vacation this year, what color couch should we get, why is Facebook down, and why did they cancel *Firefly*?

But there's one aspect of existence that hasn't changed and never will. And that's the sheer amount of effort it takes to create financial success, recognition, and the satisfaction of self-actualization.

The trials of our forebears revolved around how to stay alive. Ours revolve around how to feel alive. A thousand years ago, someone too lazy to go to "work" starved to death. Today, he gets on welfare. But is he alive? I don't think so.

It takes effort-focused, persistent, dedicated work toward a goal—to create anything of any value, whether it's a good family, a good career, a good social life, or anything else.

This is a vital life lesson that working out regularly teaches us: he or she who can confront and exert effort reaps the rewards. And the greater the efforts, the greater the rewards.

If you've ever squatted until your legs were Jell-O, you know what I'm talking about. If you've ever skimped on sleep, hangouts, or precious TV time to get your workout in, you know what I'm talking about. If you've ever filled your fridge with Tupperware full of carefully weighed meals, you know what I'm talking about.

Despite what fake gurus and pill and powder pushers say, there are no shortcuts in this lifestyle. You either do the work, or you don't. And you either transform your body, or you don't.

The rest of life is the same. I cringe every time I see someone I know hunting for shortcuts to success, secretly obsessed with avoiding effort. Gotta get more for less. Gotta work smarter, not harder. Gotta find an easier way.

It's BS.

I'm all for seizing opportunities and being clever, but no amount of genius allows you to escape this rule of effort.

I'm not the smartest person, but I can succeed because I'm willing to outwork whatever I lack intellectually. I don't care if that means 14-hour workdays and being known as the "boring guy who's always working." I don't care if that means working weekends while my friends are goofing off. I don't care about the latest TV shows, and I don't care about "taking it easy." And that's why I've gone from nothing to more than 150,000 books sold in just two years...as a self-published author.

For me, it's not about getting rich. It's not about trying to become famous. It's much more primal than that. And personal.

It's why we push ourselves for one more rep on our last set of Deadlifts, it's why we crawl out of bed after legs day happily crippled, and it's why we go to the gym to *beat the crap out of ourselves*—not to chat and take cute selfies.

It's about knowing deep down that we're tough sons of bitches. That we're wired differently from everyone else. That while we may not always win, we *never* lose because we didn't work hard enough.

PATIENCE AND LEARNING TO LOVE THE PROCESS

"Are we there yet?" a child will repeat incessantly, sick of staring at the same, rolling pastures, dreaming about arriving at Disney World.

Well, the average person pursuing a goal hasn't changed much since childhood. He fantasizes about where he wants to be and quickly grows bored with the drudgery of getting there.

This lesson is similar to the last but not the same. This one relates to breaking the obsession with instant gratification, which is basically a hallmark of our current society.

Whether it's weight loss or work, success always comes more slowly than we want. Even when it's fast, it's still too damn slow. If we let them, these feelings of restlessness, frustration, and impatience will derail us in every endeavor.

We must learn to focus on and enjoy the process of arriving at the goal. We must disabuse ourselves of the idea that satisfaction only comes from having, not doing.

This is another lesson we learn by working out regularly: we learn to appreciate the process of making slow, steady improvements that, in time, add up to major change.

There's something special about this state. It's almost Zen-like. When we stop counting on miracles or quick fixes, when we stop weighing and measuring ourselves every day wondering whether we're there yet and instead embrace the process, we fall into a calm, confident rhythm. We learn to confront time, and minor setbacks lose their power over our emotions. Progress is no longer a matter of hope. In the process we trust, and it never betrays.

So it is in the gym, it is in work and life.

For me, the completion of a work project or the fulfillment of a goal is a bittersweet moment. I'm happy to have arrived but always find myself reminiscing about the journey, almost nostalgically. There's something comforting about the process, knowing that I'm spending my time going somewhere. And I quickly stop caring about what I've achieved and long to start on something new.

When you're addicted to *the process of arriving*, not *having arrived*, you've learned this lesson well, and your life will change for the better.

YOU CAN DO MORE THAN YOU THINK

We all have forces within us that want us to fail. That tell us we're too dumb, too lazy, or too clumsy. That genuinely resent anything creative or constructive that we try to do. They can be incredibly persuasive and work tirelessly to squash us.

Some people call them resistance. Others refer to them as demons.

Well, regardless of what you call these ethereal enemies, if you want to see how effective they are, just take a good, honest look at the people around you. How many are truly confident in their abilities? How many can calmly deal with criticism or even banter? How many refrain from talking themselves up and others down?

I think it's clear that many of us are suffering from greater or lesser crises of confidence. And they hold us back in every area our lives. They convince us that it's safer to stay small, to not even try. If we let them, they make cowards of us all.

We tell ourselves otherwise, of course. We need to believe we're in control. That we choose to be this way. But we're just afraid—afraid of failure, of what others will think, and of what *we'll* think.

Well, when you work out regularly, you learn to tune out the voices. You learn to believe in yourself and in your ability to make stuff happen.

Most people think that the only boost of self-confidence that comes with exercise relates to losing weight or building muscle—to looking better. But that's not the whole picture.

When you start lifting weights, you're a weakling. You feel like Gumby, and the voices mock and ridicule you. But you keep going, and you get better. You learn to stop making excuses. You learn that you can be in control simply by stepping foot in the gym despite any head trash that tries to stop you. And by doing that, you sap them of their power.

This is an ability you gain, and it's good for a lot more than just getting a pretty physique.

Half of any battle you face in life is just showing up every day despite how you feel. That's what makes a real pro. He doesn't wait for inspiration to get to work. He doesn't bargain with himself. He puts his ass in the chair every day like he knows he should, and by doing this, he learns to master his emotions. As you learn in the gym, once you get going on something constructive, you always feel better.

When you realize that you can control your emotions through your behavior, and when you're confident enough to keep taking the right actions, you create a powerful engine for change in any area of your life.

THE BOTTOM LINE

If I've done a good job in this chapter, I think you'll agree that we should train for a lot more than merely looking or feeling better.

We should use our training to harness the power of habit, to maintain a high willingness to exert effort, to stay mentally and physically tough, to remind us of the importance of patience and consistency, and to bolster our self-confidence to face the various challenges of life.

So, let's now move on to the physical and practical, starting with how to achieve the Holy Grail of fitness: strength, aesthetics, and health.

2

ACHIEVING THE FITNESS HOLY GRAIL: STRENGTH, AESTHETICS, AND HEALTH

FOR YOUR FIRST FEW YEARS OF training, your goal is very simple: put on as much muscle and get as strong as possible.

While that may not sound very inspiring, it amounts to quite a dramatic transformation. It means gaining 30 to 40 pounds of muscle and tripling or even quadrupling your lifts across the board. People who haven't seen you for a while don't believe their eyes.

Once you've achieved this, you'll have come to like what you see in the mirror, and you won't be solely driven by the goal to look pretty—you'll love training for its own sake and thrive on the effort it takes to add another pound of muscle or another 10 pounds to the bar.

It's at this point, however, that your fitness goals should evolve.

Your ability to add mass and strength is greatly diminished, so your mentality has to change. Gone are the simple days of adding weight to the bar every week and eating everything in sight.

Don't fall into the trap of complacency where you're just showing up, moving some weight around, and going home. The reality is that as time goes on, making gains becomes harder and harder, which makes falling into a rut easier and easier.

The way to prevent this is always know exactly where you're going and why, which helps you keep your schedule, maintain the intensity of your workouts, and manage your diet.

You now have to focus on three more specific, finer points of bodybuilding and weightlifting:

1. Improving the proportions and overall aesthetics of your physique

2. Improving your strength, one rep at a time

3. Staying healthy

Fortunately, you can do all three at the same time. That's what this book is all about.

So, then, let's look at the above goals in more detail.

CREATING A MORE AESTHETIC PHYSIQUE

Aesthetics is all the Internet fitness crowd talks about these days, so I hate the word, but I'm going to run with it anyway.

What I'm referring to is simply the visual attractiveness of your body—not just raw size, but proportions and symmetry. Sometimes relatively small changes in a physique can make a big difference visually.

For instance...

- A small upper chest will tend to give your pecs a rounder, "bottom-heavy" look instead of the flatter, "armor plate" look we're after.

- The larger your arms are, the larger your shoulders need to be to compensate. Small shoulders on top of large arms create a lopsided look.

- If your shoulder-to-hip ratio is lacking (if you don't have enough of a V-taper), the more muscular your torso, the blockier you look.

- If your calves are lacking, you look like you have chicken legs when you wear shorts, regardless of how big your quads and hamstrings are.

- Unless you particularly like it this way, having small traps on a large upper body looks off. For many people, large traps immediately increase the appearance of overall muscularity, whereas small traps produce the opposite effect.

- An underdeveloped core will always leave you disappointed, regardless of how lean you get. If your abs or obliques are too small, or if you're lacking in serratus development, you'll never quite have that shredded look, even when you're in the 6 to 7% body fat range.

As you can see, you can hone in on quite a few things if you want to sculpt the ideal physique. And in the next chapter, we'll revisit this subject and show you how to pinpoint exactly what you need to improve in your physique to maximize its visual appeal.

Now, nitpicking your physique might not be your thing, and that's totally fine. Instead, you might be more interested in just maximizing strength and allowing your body to continue to add mass in the same way it has been up to this point.

Hell, some people's genetics are so good they don't need to even do much in the way of focusing on weak points—they just lift heavy and eat right, and symmetry and proportion come naturally. If that's you, high-five your parents and share the wealth by having a lot of children!

But that's pretty rare. Most people with great physiques had to carefully engineer them that way. And by the end of this book, you'll have all the tools you need to do the same.

Next, let's talk about the second goal: improving strength, one rep at a time.

GETTING STRONGER, ONE REP AT A TIME

Being strong is just plain fun.

There's a primal satisfaction that comes with being able to push, pull, and lift gargantuan amounts of weight.

Super strength doesn't come easily, however. It's built one rep at a time.

What do I mean by that?

Well, this is something I mentioned in *BLS*, but it's especially relevant as you dive into this book and its workout program.

In every workout, your goal is to beat your last workout. But beating it in terms of actual weight on the bar isn't realistic on a week-to-week basis. What is, however, is beating your previous week's reps with a given weight.

Even if it's only by one rep on one exercise, that's progress. That's how you have to view your training. Because those extra reps add up and eventually allow you to increase weight on the bar.

The *Beyond Bigger Leaner Stronger* program is built with this in mind. You won't be adding weight on a set schedule; instead, you will follow your body's lead and increase weight as you actually get stronger in your workouts. And it will make you stronger than you've ever been before.

Let's now talk about the final goal: staying healthy.

IN THE END, HEALTH IS WHAT MATTERS MOST

As an experienced lifter, you face a few unique health risks.

Drugs are one.

The "middle years" of your training can be quite discouraging if you don't know exactly what you're doing. You can spend hours and hours in the gym every week, eat "clean," and get nowhere.

This can lead to frustration and eventually desperation, and steroids might seem like the only way out.

Well, while certain types of steroids may not be as inherently dangerous as most people think, if you don't know what you're doing, you can mess yourself up for life. And even if you are well informed, you can't escape the health risks of some of the more popular drugs, and the psychological addiction can be quite powerful (any honest steroid user can attest to this).

The likelihood of injury, and the potential severity of that injury, are other risks.

Although it places a lot of strain on the body, weightlifting is quite safe…when you stick to weights you can properly handle and remain very strict on form.

How often do you see guys throwing caution to the wind, though? Stacking plates on plates for a hunchbacked Deadlift, shaking half Squat, or impossible Bench Press?

Newbies don't tend to make these types of mistakes. They are almost always perpetrated by the guy who's been hitting the gym for a few years and feels he should be lifting more, and thinks his body can handle whatever he throws at it.

Well, this behavior not only dramatically increases the risk of injury, but it also increases the risk of *serious* injury—torn muscles, ruined joints, or worse—the stuff that you have to deal with for the rest of your life.

Yet another health risk unique to the experienced lifter relates to metabolism and general well-being.

Once most guys have built some size, they finally want to get shredded. And there's a lot of really bad advice out there on how to do it.

The most common, harmful practice I come across is combining near-starvation diets with excessive exercise, which puts an unbelievable amount of stress on your body and crashes your metabolism and anabolic hormones.

"Nobody said getting ripped is easy," says the online coach prescribing the program, so the person continues. Eventually, he completely burns out and faces a severely damaged metabolism and impaired immune system, not to mention a deep feeling of disappointment.

Properly navigating your way around these risks is a major part of long-term success and fulfillment. The goal isn't to look good for a few years while ruining your body in the process but to establish a sustainable lifestyle that gives you the physique you want while improving your health and longevity.

Well, this book will help you do just that. It will show you how to safely and healthfully break through the "mediocre middle" and build an outstanding physique that you can enjoy for the rest of your life.

So, with that in mind, let's now take a closer look at how to build a great physique. Did you know that there is a fairly precise science of finding strengths and weakness in your physique? And that you can use this information to get your body to as close to "perfect" as possible?

Turn the page to learn more.

3

THE MATHEMATICS OF AESTHETICS: HOW TO BUILD THE IDEAL MALE BODY

LET'S FACE IT: A BIG REASON why many of us work out every day is to look as awesome as possible.

And to us, that doesn't mean looking like a hulking bodybuilder. Sure, it means being muscular, but it also means having a lean, proportional physique that still looks athletic—the type of body that other men wish they had and women swoon over, not frown at.

This is what we mean when we talk about acquiring an *aesthetic* physique: a body that just looks damn good.

You know it when you see it: broad shoulders with bulging biceps and triceps extending below; a big, flat chest on top of a clear V-taper that ends with a narrow waist and defined core; and developed, striated legs that end in calves like biceps. And all wrapped in very little fat, giving it all a tight, hard look.

Although bodybuilding today is all about packing on freakish amounts of mass, it used to place an emphasis on aesthetics. For example, look at the legendary Steve Reeves, whose physique is attainable naturally.

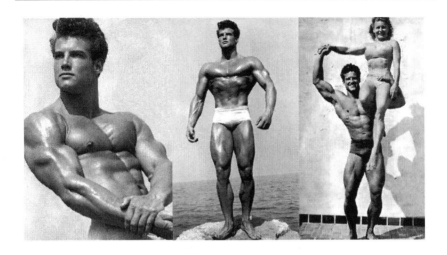

Reeves would be considered a scrawny weakling by today's professional bodybuilding standards, but damn, he looked good, right?

Well, it turns out that there's a mathematical symmetry underlying a physique like his, which we'll talk more about in a minute.

How do we get there, though?

Workouts of the week for a massive chest and shredded arms won't cut it. It requires a deeper understanding of what exactly creates that look and what you need to do with your body to get there.

And it doesn't depend on genetics either. While we may not have Reeves's genetics, we can achieve the same types of proportions and improve the overall look of our physiques.

No, we can't make our bodies carbon copies of our physical role models because muscle shape, length, and insertion points vary from person to person, but we can all build bodies that look awesome.

Building an aesthetic physique is formulaic, and anyone can do it.

In this chapter, I'm going to show you how to take stock of your current physique and determine which parts need work to achieve the type of physique that makes people say "wow."

Let's start with the theory of ideal physical size and proportions, which is more of a science than many people realize. In fact, it has its roots in a fascinating ratio underlying much of the beauty and symmetry we find in nature...

THE GOLDEN RATIO AND THE BODY

In the first century B.C., at the dawn of the Roman imperial age, the architect Marcus Vitruvius published one of the most important sources of modern knowledge of Roman building methods, planning, and design. It covers almost every aspect of Roman architecture, from town planning, to building materials, to the construction of temples, civil and domestic buildings, pavements, aqueducts, and more.

Vitruvius's publication also describes what he felt were the ideal human proportions, and he thought that sacred temples should conform to these proportions. In fact, he believed that the human body reflected the hidden geometry of the universe and thus was a microcosmic representation of the physical realm.

Sound far-fetched to you? Probably so to most average intellectuals, but not to Leonardo da Vinci.

Over 1,500 years later, sometime around 1487, da Vinci drew the human figure in accordance with Vitruvius's observations and named it the *Vitruvian Man*. He had the same fascination with human anatomy as Vitruvius: he believed that, in his own words, "man is a model of the world."

The answer to that enigmatic statement lies in what's known as the *divine proportion* or *Golden Ratio*. For more than 2,000 years, esteemed mathematicians and scientists have studied, pondered, and debated this ratio and its ubiquity in nature, mathematics, architecture, and art.

So, what is this ratio? Euclid first defined it in *Elements*, published in 300 B.C. The concept is simple: two quantities are in the Golden Ratio if the ratio of the sum of the quantities to the larger quantity is equal to the ratio of the larger quantity to the smaller one.

Visually, it looks like this:

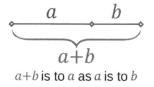

$a+b$ is to a as a is to b

And numerically, it's expressed like this: 1:1.618 (1 to 1.618). In the case of the above image, b is 1 unit long, and a is 1.618 units long.

Now, the fascinating thing about the Golden Ratio is its plausibility as a natural law. Scientists have found its expression in the arrangement of branches along the stems of plants and in the veins of leaves, in the skeletons of animals and the disposition of their veins and nerves, and in the composition of chemical compounds and the geometry of crystals. Researchers have recently reported the ratio present even at the atomic level.

Nowhere is the Golden Ratio more exemplified than in the human body, however, as da Vinci knew so long ago. In fact, he found that the more the body reflected this proportion, the more beautiful it was.

The human face, for instance, abounds with examples of the Golden Ratio. The head forms a golden rectangle with the eyes at its midpoint. The mouth and nose are each placed at golden distances between the eyes and the bottom of the chin. The spatial relationship of the teeth and the construction of the ear each reflect the ratio too.

Further, the Golden Ratio is found in the overall proportions of the human body: the different lengths of the finger bones, the makeup of the feet and toes, and even the structure of DNA.

When various parts of the body are in the Golden Ratio to others, a beautiful symmetry and proportion are created. Artists have known this for centuries. Modern plastic surgeons and cosmetic dentists use this knowledge to create beautiful faces and mouths.

When we apply the Golden Ratio to our purposes, we find that by adjusting the size of various body parts in relation to others, we're able to immediately improve visual attractiveness.

There are many examples of how the Golden Ratio points the way to an aesthetic physique, and instead of breaking it down piece by piece, we're going to use a few shortcuts that relate to measuring and comparing certain parts of your body.

ACHIEVING THE "GRECIAN IDEAL"

The ancient Greeks were known for their portrayal of what they felt was the ideal male physique. Statues often portrayed men with small waists; broad, muscular shoulders; and developed, defined legs.

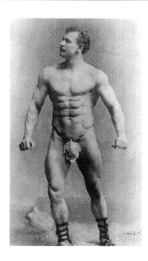

Eugen Sandow *(above)*, the legendary strongman from the late 1800s and "father of bodybuilding," was renowned for his resemblance to the classical Greek and Roman sculptures. It was no accident.

Sandow measured the statues in museums and found that certain proportions remained constant (and as you now know, these proportions have their roots in the Golden Ratio).

This led to the development of the "Grecian Ideal" as a formula for building the perfect physique, and Sandow's goal was to embody it.

Sandow's body and principles served as the model for future bodybuilders who became known for their beautifully balanced physiques, like Steve Reeves, Frank Zane, Danny Padilla, Serge Nubret, Bob Paris, and Arnold Schwarzenegger.

So, what are these proportions? How can we too look like the Greek gods?

Well, it starts with establishing reference points—parts of the body whose sizes will determine how large other parts must be to achieve an overall aesthetic physique. Some of these reference points, such as the wrist and knee, don't change in size as you age or as your conditioning changes. Others, such as the waist, do.

For example, by measuring your wrist size, you can determine how large your upper arms should be, and from that measurement how large your neck and calves should be. Your knee size determines how large your upper leg should be, and your waist size tells you how broad your chest and shoulders should be.

Let's now look at the formula for acquiring the "perfect" physique:

Your flexed arms should be 150% larger than the circumference of your non-dominant wrist (wrist measurement x 2.5)

Measure the smallest part of your wrist with a measuring tape, and measure the largest part of your flexed arm (the peak of your bicep and middle of your triceps).

It's worth mentioning that some people will say that such formulas apply to an unflexed arm, but I disagree. My wrists are 7 inches. My arms are just over 17 inches flexed and 14.5 inches unflexed, and they almost look too large. Getting them up to 17 inches unflexed and 20+ inches flexed would look absolutely ridiculous.

Even if you lack a prominent bicep peak, stick with flexed measurements.

Your flexed calves should match your flexed arms

The general rule is your calves should match your arms, and if we're talking flexed arms, then we should be talking flexed calves.

You measure this by flexing your calf (raising your heel off the ground) and wrapping a measuring tape around the largest part.

Your shoulder circumference should measure 1.618 times larger than your waist (waist x 1.618)

You measure your waist by circling it with a measuring tape (sort of like a belt would) at your natural waistline, which is located above your belly button and below your ribcage. Don't suck in your stomach.

You measure your shoulder circumference as follows:

Stand upright with your arms comfortably at your sides (no flaring your elbows or spreading your lats), and have a friend wrap a measuring tape around your shoulders and chest at its widest point. This is usually right around the top of your armpits.

Your chest circumference should be 550% larger than the circumference of your non-dominant wrist (wrist measurement x 6.5)

To take your chest measurement, stand upright with your arms comfortably at your sides (no flaring your elbows or spreading your lats). Have a friend place a measuring tape at the fullest part of one of your pecs and wrap it around your upper body, under your armpits, across your shoulder blades, and back to the starting point.

There are other ways to reach the ideal chest measurement, but this is the easiest and most reliable.

Your upper leg circumference should be 75% larger than your knee circumference (knee measurement x 1.75)

To measure your knee circumference, place the measuring tape at the tip of your kneecap and wrap around.

To get your upper leg measurement, wrap a measuring tape around the biggest part of your thigh and hamstring. This can vary from person to person, depending on how the muscles develop.

All right then. Are you ready to see how you measure up?

COMPARING YOUR PHYSIQUE TO THE IDEAL PHYSIQUE

Tape measuring each part of your body is the most accurate method, and while any old tape measure will do, I like a specific one made just for this purpose (you'll find it in the bonus report to this book).

Another important point to consider is your body fat percentage. If you're carrying excess fat, your measurements will be skewed, with some affected more than others (your waist, for example, will be greatly affected, but your calves will not).

So if you want to truly know what needs improving, you need to get lean first.

How lean?

That's up to you, but I would say no higher than 10% body fat. Personally, I like to maintain a leaner look than that (7 to 8%), and thus that's the point from which I base all readings.

Let's now get to the measuring, starting with your current status.

Take and record the following measurements (do both sides of your body where applicable so you can assess symmetry):

- Your non-dominant wrist circumference

- Your arms

- Your shoulder circumference

- Your chest circumference

- Your waist

- Your upper legs

- Your knees

- Your calves

Once you know these measurements, you can simply compare them against the formula given earlier.

For example, here are my current measurements, at 7% body fat compared to my ideal numbers:

Current Measurements	Ideal Measurements
7-inch wrist	N/A
17-inch arms	17.5-inch arms
51-inch shoulder circumference	52-inch shoulder circumference
43-inch chest circumference	45.5-inch chest circumference
32-inch waist	N/A
24-inch upper legs	25-inch upper legs
14-inch knee	N/A
15.5-inch calves	17.5-inch calves

According to the above, I need to increase my shoulder, chest, upper leg, and calf measurements, and I completely agree. My shoulders are a bit small for my arm size, my chest is okay but I need more lats (which will expand my chest measurement), my upper legs are playing catch-up (I neglected them for my first several years of weightlifting), and my calves definitely need some size.

And my training reflects these goals. I train shoulders twice per week and calves three times per week, and I do extra work on my quads on legs day and lats on back day. (We'll talk more about exactly how to train weak points in a later chapter.)

YOUR TURN

Take your measurements and see where you're strong and where you're lacking, and I bet you'll agree. And even if you don't want to match the numbers exactly—maybe you'd prefer your arms or upper legs an inch smaller or larger—it helps point you in the right direction.

Now, once you know what needs work, the next question is how you do it in terms of diet and training.

Well, we'll talk more about these things soon, but first, I want to take a few minutes to talk about the subject of natural muscle growth.

Why?

Because before you start comparing your measurements to other very unnatural "natural" bodybuilders online and feel completely inadequate or worry that your numbers will never reach the ideal proportions laid out in this chapter, I want you to understand how much muscle you can build naturally and how long it takes.

4

HOW MUCH MUSCLE CAN YOU BUILD NATURALLY, AND HOW QUICKLY?

I AM OFTEN ASKED HOW MUCH muscle one can build naturally. That is, how can we determine our genetic potential in terms of building muscle? How big can we get without taking drugs?

If you poke around on the 'Net, you'll find a ton of conflicting opinions. Some people feel that genetics can prevent you from ever looking good, while others believe that you can accomplish anything if you work hard enough at it.

Who's right?

Neither. The truth is somewhere in the middle.

MUSCLE BUILDING AND GENETIC POTENTIAL

The first thing you should know is there isn't any way to know for sure what your genetic potential is when it comes to building muscle. While you'll never be able to gain 100 pounds of lean mass naturally, it's impossible to say with complete accuracy how big you'll be able to get.

That said, worrying about such matters before you have a few years of proper lifting and eating under your belt is pointless in my opinion. If you're new to lifting, don't even give a second thought to whether you'll be able to build enough muscle, build it quickly enough, have the right proportions, etc. This can lead to unrealistic expectations and an early mental defeat.

The ultimate reality is that you are going to train hard, eat right, and let your body develop as it will. While we don't all have the genetics to be top-tier bodybuilders, any of us can build a strong, muscular, healthy body that we're proud of, and that's what it's all about in the end.

So, then, how much muscle can we hope to build naturally?

HOW MUCH MUSCLE YOU CAN BUILD NATURALLY?

Unfortunately, I don't know of any studies that definitively answer this question, which is why there are so many opinions and broscience theories out there.

However, a few of the top coaches and minds in the fitness world—Lyle McDonald, Alan Aragon, and Martin Berkhan—have developed some guidelines.

These guys have collectively worked with hundreds of elite bodybuilders and athletes and speak from not just an incredibly in-depth understanding of the body but also a wealth of real-world practice and results.

Let's look at what they have to say, and then I'll share my thoughts and experiences.

Lyle McDonald's Answer

Mr. McDonald keeps his model very simple. (And as a sidenote, this applies to men. Mr. McDonald says women should expect about half of these numbers.):

YEARS OF PROPER TRAINING	POTENTIAL MUSCLE GAINS
1	20 to 25 pounds
2	10 to 12 pounds
3	5 to 6 pounds
4+	2 to 3 pounds

According to Mr. McDonald, both age and starting condition will affect this number. Older guys will gain less than younger ones, and underweight guys can gain more than this. And some people can just build more or less muscle due to other factors like hormones, genetics, and lifestyle.

As you can see, Mr. McDonald says that you're looking at 40 to 50 pounds of muscle you can gain in your first 4 to 5 years, and the gains are negligible from there on out.

Also notice that it's years of *proper* training, not just training. Mr. McDonald said that someone who has been lifting improperly for several years has the potential to make "year 1" gains when he starts training properly. (And if you've read *BLS*, you know what is meant by proper and improper training.)

Alan Aragon's Answer

Mr. Aragon's model addresses the issue differently, but the numbers come out to be about the same.

CATEGORY	RATE OF MUSCLE GROWTH
Beginner	1 to 1.5% of total body weight per month
Intermediate	0.5 to 1% of total body weight per month
Advanced	0.25 to 0.5% of total body weight per month

According to Mr. Aragon's formula, a 150 lb. beginner could gain about 1.5 to 2.25 pounds of muscle per month, or 18 to 27 pounds in year 1.

Once he hits year 2, he's an intermediate lifter weighing in at 170 pounds (let's say) and could gain 0.85 to 1.7 pounds of muscle per month, or 10 to 20 pounds in year 2.

By year 3, he's an advanced lifter at, let's say, 190 pounds and is capable of gaining 5 to 10 pounds of muscle that year. His potential gains diminish from this point on.

Martin Berkhan's Answer

Mr. Berkhan developed his formula after observing and coaching scores of professional bodybuilding competitors, and it's very simple:

Height in centimeters – 100 = Upper weight limit in kg in contest shape (4 to 5% body fat)

Here's how this pans out for a few heights and weights:

HEIGHT	WEIGHT AT 5% BODY FAT	WEIGHT AT 10% BODY FAT	TOTAL MUSCLE MASS
5'8"	160 lbs.	170 lbs.	153 lbs.
5'10"	171 lbs.	180 lbs.	162 lbs.
6'	182 lbs.	192 lbs.	173 lbs.

To calculate numbers for other heights, multiply the inches by 2.54 to get centimeters. Then subtract 100 for your maximum weight in kilograms at 5% body fat. Multiply this number by 2.2 to get pounds .

MY THOUGHTS AND EXPERIENCES

This subject can lead to some extremely heated debates in weightlifting/bodybuilding circles.

Some people dismiss such formulas as useless because they don't take into account drive, work ethic, and consistency. I disagree. My experience in my own training and coaching hundreds of others aligns with the above guidelines.

I started at 155 pounds, and here's a shot of me at 175 pounds, after about 1.5 years of IMPROPER training:

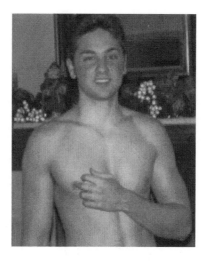

I did things well enough to ride my newbie gains, which added up to about 20 pounds in that period, with maybe 15 pounds of it being muscle—not too good. And as you can see, I am not a genetic freak by any means. I was just a normal ecto-meso.

This shot of me you saw earlier was after 6 to 7 years of improper training (I was working exclusively in the 10 to 12 rep range, was doing a lot of isolation work, wasn't squatting or deadlifting every week, had no idea what to do with diet beyond eating a lot, and so forth):

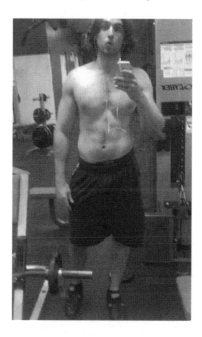

I weighed around 200 pounds here, at about 17% body fat. In the 5 to 6 years that ensued between these first two pictures, I had gained a measly 10 to 15 pounds of muscle. Pretty bad considering how much time I had put in.

Within a year or so of that last picture, I decided to truly educate myself. And in the few years that have passed since then, I've radically transformed my body.

Here's a recent shot of me at 184 pounds and about 6% body fat:

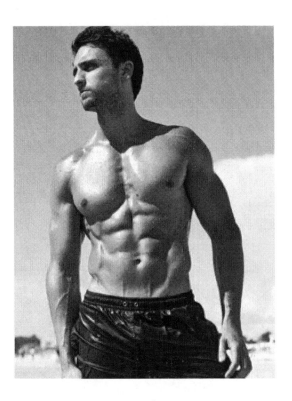

If we compare the gains I made in just a few years against the above formulas, we see that I've done VERY well for being an advanced lifter. But that's only because I made about half the gains I should've made in my first 6 to 7 years of training.

I'm now approaching my genetic potential (according to the above formulas, I have maybe 10 more pounds of muscle I can gain, and it will take several years), but I could've reached my current point several years ago had I been training and eating properly.

It's also worth mentioning that my experience coaching hundreds of guys verifies my own experiences. You can gain a LOT of muscle in your first 3 years of training if you do it right. It starts to slow down at that point. And if you've been training improperly for several years, you can make startling gains by doing it right.

DON'T DISCOURAGE YOURSELF—JUST TRAIN HARD AND EAT RIGHT, AND THE RESULTS WILL COME

Some people look to professional bodybuilders, who step on stage at 270+ pounds and shredded, and feel deflated when they're told that they'll never be much bigger than 190 pounds in contest shape.

Well, the reality is 190 pounds at 5 to 7% is huge by normal standards. You're fitness cover model material. Girls will love you, and guys will want to be you (cheesy, sorry).

Unless you're trying to reach freak status, you can achieve the look you want naturally.

Just know that it takes several years of hard work, but also that between *BLS* and this book, you have everything you need to get there.

In the next chapter, we're going to dive into the real meat and potatoes of the theory behind most advanced training programs, including the *Beyond Bigger Leaner Stronger* program—the science of "periodization," as it's known.

5

AN INTRODUCTION TO ADVANCED TRAINING PRINCIPLES: THE SCIENCE OF PROPER PERIODIZATION

IF YOU'VE PUT IN YOUR TIME on my *BLS* program, you know how effective heavy, compound weightlifting is.

It builds muscle and strength, and *fast*. It is, in my opinion, the absolute best way to spend your first 1 to 2 years of lifting. It will deliver the maximum amount of natural muscle growth possible in that time (20 to 40 pounds) and will build a solid foundation of all-around strength and power.

Once you've achieved that, however, you can begin to "periodize" your training. "Periodization" is a just a fancy word that refers to methodical variations in training, such as changes in workout volume (number of sets performed), intensity (percentage of one-rep max, or *1RM*, lifted), exercises performed, rest times, etc.

What type of periodization am I talking about here? Well, as you'll see, the primary difference between the workouts in this book and the *BLS* workouts is the inclusion of lower- and higher-rep sets.

Why would you want to do this? Why not just continue performing all sets in the 4 to 6 rep range?

Well, you can't go *wrong* by doing sticking with this rep range—you will continue to make gains—but you should consider a couple of things:

1. Some people simply get bored of doing the same type of training

for long periods, and this mental staleness leads to physical staleness, which manifests in the gym and stunts progress.

2. Different factors contribute to maximal growth, each of which is best addressed by different rep ranges. (We'll talk about this in detail in a minute.)

The training method espoused in the *Beyond Bigger Leaner Stronger* program is known as "power bodybuilding," because it combines the training principles of powerlifting and traditional bodybuilding, and it's been around for at least two decades.

Its effectiveness can be seen in the simple fact that the biggest bodybuilders are often the strongest. This correlation was particularly true before the use of insulin and growth hormone became prevalent in the bodybuilding world.

(All the major steroids available to today's bodybuilders were also available to the bodybuilders of Arnold Schwarzenegger's time, but insulin and growth hormone were not used in the '70s. Once these two drugs hit the scene, they enabled bodybuilders to go from the "big but aesthetic" look that Arnie personified to the "holy s*&% you're a monster" look of today.)

Now, before we get into the nuts and bolts of the *Beyond Bigger Leaner Stronger* program, I want to briefly revisit the never-ending debate as to which is best for building muscle—low reps, heavy weight, or high-reps, low weight?

I probably don't have to sell you on the importance of heaving lifting and progressive overload, as you've experienced firsthand its effectiveness with the *BLS* program. But I want to give you a little insight as to why I'm recommending periodization in the *Beyond Bigger Leaner Stronger* program.

Let's start with a deeper look at the physiology of muscle tissue and of how it grows bigger and stronger.

NOT ALL MUSCLE FIBERS ARE EQUAL

Muscle tissue is a complex structure, with bundles of long strands of muscle cells (known as fibers) sheathed in a thick band of connective tissue known as a perimysium. Here's how it looks:

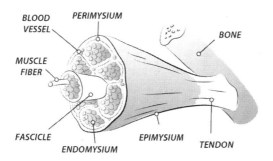

Now, these individual muscle fibers come in different types. There are three major divisions:

1. Type I

2. Type IIa

3. Type IIx

Type I muscle fibers, also known as slow-twitch muscle fibers, have the lowest potential for growth and force output.[3] However, they are dense with capillaries and rich in mitochondria and myoglobin, which makes them resistant to fatigue.

Type II fibers, also known as fast-twitch muscle fibers, both a and x, have a much higher potential for growth and force output than Type I fibers, but they fatigue quickly.[4] In bodybuilding, we are primarily concerned with these types of fibers.

Now, we all have varying numbers of Type I and Type II fibers in our bodies, and the ratios are heavily influenced by how we use our muscles.[5] If we did a lot of long-distance running, we would develop more Type I fibers in our legs than Type II. If we did a lot of heavy squatting, we would develop more Type II fibers.

The same goes for rep schemes in weightlifting. A simple, but not incorrect, way to look at it is training in the 4 to 6 rep range mainly hits Type IIx fibers, the 10 to 12 rep range hits Type IIa, and the 30 to 40+ rep range hits Type I fibers.[6]

Simple enough. Let's now move on to the physiology of muscle growth and how it's affected by different types of training.

HOW TO STIMULATE MUSCLE GROWTH

Three primary factors are involved in stimulating muscle growth:[7]

1. Progressive tension overload

2. Muscle damage

3. Cellular fatigue

Progressive tension is, in my opinion (and the opinion of quite a few experts much smarter than me), the most important of the three.[8] It refers to progressively increasing tension levels in the muscle fibers over time: that is, lifting progressively heavier and heavier weights.

Muscle damage refers to just that—actual damage caused to the muscle fibers by high levels of tension. This damage necessitates repair, and if the body is provided with proper nutrition and rest, it will grow the fibers to better deal with future stimuli.

Cellular fatigue refers to pushing muscle fibers to their metabolic limits through the repetition of actions to muscular failure. This is known as subjecting cells to "metabolic stress."

You can think of these three factors as separate growth pathways. That is, each can be targeted in training, and each stimulate hypertrophy to a greater or lesser degree.

It may have already occurred to you, but this is why natural weightlifters who focus on high-rep lifting, with little to no heavy lifting that gets progressively heavier over time, fail to make any noticeable gains.

They are inducing a lot of cellular fatigue, especially if they do supersets, dropsets, and other fancy rep schemes, with some resulting muscle damage, but in the absence of progressive tension overload, muscle growth is very slow.

These "pump trainers" also often focus on isolation exercises, further reducing the effectiveness of their workouts (the sheer number of muscle fibers you activate in a workout greatly affects overall growth[9]).

This is why my *BLS* program is the complete opposite: it's built around heavy, compound lifting that gets heavier over time and that targets Type II fibers, which can grow big and strong quickly.

And, as you'll see, the *Beyond Bigger Leaner Stronger* program is built around the *BLS* style of weightlifting but with the introduction of extremely heavy sets for maximum overload as well as lighter sets for targeting Type IIx fibers and induce metabolic stress.

But, before we dive more into that, let's review another aspect of muscle growth: the two ways muscles grow larger and how they relate to your training.

THE TWO TYPES OF MUSCLE GROWTH

Although we don't fully understand the mechanisms just yet, it's generally accepted that there are two types of hypertrophy (muscle growth):

1. Myofibrillar hypertrophy

2. Sarcoplasmic hypertrophy[10]

Myofibrillar hypertrophy refers to an actual increase in size of the muscle fibers and sarcoplasmic hypertrophy to an increase in the volume of the fluid, non-contractile components of the muscle (glycogen, water, minerals, etc.).

If we look at rep ranges on a continuum going from very heavy weight for one rep to very light weights for 40+ reps, the following generally holds true:

Heavier lifting preferentially induces myofibrillar growth, and lighter lifting sarcoplasmic growth. Heavier lifting does result in some sarcoplasmic growth[11][12] and lighter lifting some myofibrillar growth, but the former induces more myofibrillar than sarcoplasmic, and the latter vice versa.

This too sheds some light on another big downside to working exclusively in the 10 to 12 rep range and up: you're inducing more sarcoplasmic growth than myofibrillar, and the result is that puffy type of muscle that noticeably deflates after several days of rest.

I used to train in the 10 to 12 rep range with a lot of supersets, drop sets, and giant sets, and I always hated the inflation-deflation cycle. I would train my chest on Monday and look good for a few days but then wonder where it went come Saturday.

I now have several years of heavy (myofibrillar) lifting under my belt and have built a foundation of strong, dense muscle that just doesn't deflate. I can take 1 or 2 weeks off from training and lose maybe 5% of my visual size, and I retain strength surprisingly well.

Furthermore, focusing on sarcoplasmic growth fails to build any real strength, so you stay relatively weak, even if you have some size. Focusing on myofibrillar growth, on the other hand, can greatly increase your strength.

Now, don't think that sarcoplasmic growth is worthless. It has a place in an advanced weightlifter's routine, but it should not be the focus. But we'll talk more about that in a minute.

The next bit of physiology I want to discuss before laying out the *Beyond Bigger Leaner Stronger* routine is how muscles get stronger.

HOW MUSCLES GET STRONGER

There are two ways for your muscles to produce force:

1. Recruit more muscle fibers[13]

2. Fire muscle fibers more forcefully[14]

The first is exactly what it sounds like: there are so many individual fibers in a muscle, and the more that are recruited to contract, the more force can be produced.

The second refers to how quickly the body can send electrical signals to the muscle fibers, and the better it can do this, the more forcefully the muscle fibers can contract.

An increase in strength is simply an increase in the number of muscle fibers available for recruitment (bigger muscles), an increase in the existing fibers' ability to fire, or both.

3. This, by the way, is why people can get stronger without getting bigger: neuromuscular adaptations in existing muscle fibers can improve their ability to contract without the addition of new fibers.[15] We see this in Olympic lifters, for example.

Such adaptations can only take you so far, however—once the existing fibers are "maxed out" in terms of neuromuscular efficiency, you must add more fibers to continue getting stronger. And to do this, you have to focus on increasing the amount of tension in muscles (progressive overload with heavier and heavier weights).

The bottom line is if strength stalls for extended periods, so does progressive overload and thus myofibrillar hypertrophy, and that's the end of any real progress in terms of muscle size.

This is why all good natural bodybuilding programs have as a primary goal to increase strength and primarily use heavy weightlifting (80% to 95% of 1RM) to accomplish this.

Some programs, like my *BLS* program, focus almost exclusively on the 4 to 6 rep range and are extremely effective in building both size and strength. Gaining 20 to 25 pounds of muscle (not just weight, but muscle) in year 1 and half of that in year 2 is common for *BLS* trainees.

Now, you might be wondering how such gains are possible if guys are only working in the 4 to 6 rep range. How can they build so much muscle without any pure strength training (1 to 3 reps) or sarcoplasmic training (10 to 12 reps or higher)?

Well, there are three main reasons:

1. The volume of the workouts is optimal for inducing enough muscle damage without overtraining. (More on this soon.)

2. The 4 to 6 rep set (done with about 85% of your 1RM) is a training "sweet spot" that induces both neurological adaptations that increase strength and high levels of muscle tension and damage that increase size.

3. The program has you increase weight once you reach 6 reps, which ensures that the muscles are being progressively overloaded week after week.

The bottom line is you can't go wrong sticking to the *BLS* program for years or even decades. So long as you stick to the program's protocols and ensure you're eating correctly, you will continue to make gains.

That said, once you've followed the program for 1.5 to 2 years, you'll have brought your body to a point where you can squeeze more out of it in terms of strength and hypertrophy gains. And that's where the *Beyond Bigger Leaner Stronger* program comes in. It's an evolution of *BLS*, and it's for advanced weightlifters.

Why is it only for advanced weightlifters? And what does that mean exactly? Carry on to find out.

6

HOW AND WHEN TO PERIODIZE YOUR TRAINING

YOU'VE PROBABLY CORRECTLY CONCLUDED THAT A proper periodization routine has you hitting all three pathways of hypertrophy[16]:

1. Progressive tension overload

2. Muscle damage

3. Metabolic stress/cellular fatigue

And as you know, this is accomplished by working in different rep ranges, ranging from 1 to 3 to 10 to 12 and possibly even beyond. By doing this, your training runs your body through the gamut of stimuli for both strength and hypertrophy.

Pure strength training has you working in the 1 to 3 rep range, and it primarily stimulates neurological adaptations.

Bodybuilding generally begins in the 4 to 6 rep range, which is known as a "power bodybuilding" rep range.

The 6 to 8 rep range works similar to the 4 to 6 range in terms of stimulating myofibrillar growth but with less emphasis on increasing strength and the addition of some sarcoplasmic growth.

The type of bodybuilding that's taught in most magazines falls in the 10 to 12 rep range and above (this includes things like drop sets and giant sets that have you doing 30+ reps per set).

Now, the question is how do you properly combine these different rep ranges to optimally stimulate both strength and hypertrophy?

Well, before we get into that, I want to address an important point: when you should start periodizing your training.

I've already said a few times that I believe a newbie should follow the *BLS* program for at least 1.5 to 2 years before moving on to the program I'm going to lay out in this book. There are several reasons for this:

1. The *Beyond Bigger Leaner Stronger* program requires exceptional conditioning both in terms of muscle strength and endurance to avoid overtraining. If a newbie were to start with this program, it's likely that he would find it extraordinarily hard and wind up burned out within one or two mesocycles.

2. To derive maximum benefits from both the Power and Sarcoplasmic Hypertrophy Sets, you need to be able to move large amounts of weight with good form. This is especially true with the Sarcoplasmic Sets—if you're not yet strong enough to lift heavy weights for 8 to 10 reps, it's not a very effective rep range. One of the worst things weak weightlifters can do is focus exclusively on higher-rep work. This is the best way to spin your wheels, making little to no gains beyond big pumps that disappear after a few days.

3. If you're new to weightlifting, 1 to 2 years of *BLS* will give you 25 to 35 pounds of muscle growth, with an emphasis on myofibrillar growth (which is far more important than sarcoplasmic growth when you're new). It builds a solid foundation of size and strength. The latter point (building strength) is an often-neglected part of many periodization programs, but it's vitally important because stimulating myofibrillar growth requires a certain amount of muscle tension, fatigue, and damage. To accomplish this, you must be able to lift heavy weights for moderate-to-high numbers of reps, and this requires you to be *strong*.

So, please heed my advice if you're new to weightlifting and start with *BLS*. Give it at least 1 to 1.5 years before moving on to this program. That way, you'll be coming in with enough strength to benefit from both the higher- and lower-rep work included in *Beyond Bigger Leaner Stronger* program.

If you're not new to weightlifting but aren't sure if you should start here or with *BLS*, let's keep it simple. If you can do the following, you're ready to start *Beyond Bigger Leaner Stronger*. If you can't, you should use *BLS* to get there.

Squat: 1.75 x body weight for 4 to 6 reps

Deadlift: 1.75 x body weight for 4 to 6 reps

Bench Press: 1.35 x body weight for 4 to 6 reps

Seated Military Press: 1 x body weight for 4 to 6 reps

If you can do the above, then you are strong enough to benefit from a periodized program. If you can't, then I highly recommend you get there before starting such a program.

All right then, let's now move on to what periodization models are and why we use them for *Beyond Bigger Leaner Stronger*.

A DISCUSSION OF PERIODIZATION MODELS

There are three distinct periodization models:

1. Linear periodization

2. Nonlinear periodization

3. Concurrent periodization

Linear periodization is probably the most common, and it's very simple: it starts a with period of high volume of low-intensity exercise and works gradually toward a low volume of high-intensity exercise, or vice versa.

Over the course of several months, a simple linear periodization program might have you move from training in the 12 to 15 rep range to 10 to 12 reps, to 8 to 10 reps, to 6 to 8 reps, and so on, all the way down to focusing on doubles and singles.

Another common linear periodization model found in bodybuilding is an 8-week cycle that begins with 2 weeks of submaximal effort, followed by 6 weeks of maximum-intensity training.

Now, the problem with many mainstream linear periodization programs is this: when you train in just one rep range for too long, you're building up one biomechanical capacity (muscle endurance with higher reps, pure strength with lower reps, etc.) but detraining (losing performance) in others[17].

For example, if someone did pure strength training (1 to 3 reps) for 2 to 3 months, he would find his muscle endurance has decreased in that time. Then, after 2 to 3 months of 10 to 12 rep training, his muscle endurance would be much better, but he would find his strength has decreased.

Similarly, if someone did a power bodybuilding program like *BLS* (built around the 4 to 6 rep range) for several months, it's very likely that he would lose muscle size if he then did pure strength training for a few months.

One way to overcome this limitation is to use shorter periods (2 to 3 weeks, for instance) or to use *nonlinear periodization.*

Nonlinear periodization uses shorter periods, and good programs entail 2 to 3 weeks of focusing on training in a certain rep range while training the others at a maintenance level. Such a program might look like this:

- 2 to 3 weeks of focusing on 10 to 12 reps, with maintenance work for 1 to 3 and 4 to 6 rep ranges

- 2 to 3 weeks of focusing on 4 to 6 reps, with maintenance work for 1 to 3 and 10 to 12 rep ranges

- 2 to 3 weeks of focusing on 1 to 3 reps, with maintenance work for 4 to 6 and 10 to 12 rep ranges

And so forth.

I believe that nonlinear periodization is superior to linear, but neither is my choice for *Beyond Bigger Leaner Stronger.* In this program, you're going to do something known as concurrent periodization.

Concurrent periodization has you train each biomechanical capacity (rep range) in each workout. This method was developed in Russia and is touted by many strength and bodybuilding experts (such as Louie Simmons of Westside Barbell fame) as the optimal way to periodize your training. Here's how such a workout might look:

Sets 1 to 3: 1 to 3 rep range

Sets 4 to 7: 4 to 6 rep range
Sets 8 to 10: 10 to 12 rep range
Sets 11 and 12: 20 to 30 rep range

In fact, this is very similar to the *Beyond Bigger Leaner Stronger* program setup, which we're finally ready to review!

7

THE BEYOND BIGGER LEANER STRONGER TRAINING PROGRAM

WE'VE FINALLY GOTTEN TO THE HEART of the training advice in this book: the *Beyond Bigger Leaner Stronger* training program.

The program is periodized in such a way that you will be able to continue to build your strength and maximize muscle growth.

Most of your workouts will include pure strength training, will focus on the 4 to 6 rep range that works so well, and will include some higher-rep work to induce sarcoplasmic hypertrophy and metabolic stress.

The workouts will last 45 to 60 minutes.

Your primary goal will be to add weight to the bar over time. Now that your "newbie gains" are behind you, continuing to progressively overload your muscles is more important than ever.

The exercises will look familiar if you're coming from my *BLS* program: you will do a lot of compound lifting, with some isolation work to round out your overall development.

Training frequency will remain the same as *BLS* (3 to 5 days of lifting per week), with an optional sixth workout to target weak points in your physique.

You will train in 6-week cycles, which end with a week off the weights or a Deload Week, depending on how you're feeling.

Cardio will be optional, depending on what you're doing with your diet.

That's the summary. Let's now dive into the details.

BEYOND BIGGER LEANER STRONGER PERIODIZATION

A common mistake trainers make with periodization is they simply try to do too much in each workout. You can't put equal emphasis on each major rep range without creating a workout that has you in the gym for 2+ hours, beating yourself into a pulp. This works very well with chemically enhanced weightlifters, but does not work well for us natural folk.

Proper periodization routines emphasize one rep range (and thus biomechanical capacity) over others. The *Beyond Bigger Leaner Stronger* program emphasizes the familiar rep range of 4 to 6, which calls for using about 85% of your 1RM and includes lower- and higher-rep work to supplement it.

As covered in the previous chapter, this 4 to 6 rep range delivers an impressive blend of strength gains and myofibrillar hypertrophy, and this is why it's the focus of the program.

The extremely heavy lifting that you will do will help improve the neurological function of your muscles, which will in turn enable you to lift more weight in the other rep ranges, and the lighter lifting will increase muscle endurance and stimulate sarcoplasmic hypertrophy.

So, let's now look at exactly how the routine works, starting with the mesocycle layout.

THE BEYOND BIGGER LEANER STRONGER MESOCYCLE

Mesocycle is a fancy sports training term that refers to a training phase that lasts 2 to 6 weeks.

The *Beyond Bigger Leaner Stronger* mesocycle lasts 6 weeks, and here's how it breaks down:

Weeks 1 to 4
Normal Weeks

Week 5:
Power Week

Week 6:
Deload or Rest Week

The focus of the Normal Week is myofibrillar growth with supplementary work for pure strength and sarcoplasmic hypertrophy.

The focus of the Power Week is pure strength with supplementary work for myofibrillar and sarcoplasmic growth.

The Deload or Rest Week is included to give your body a break.

Now, to understand what these weeks will entail, let's look at the five types of sets that you will be doing in your workouts:

1. Warm-Up Sets

2. Power Sets

3. One-Rep Max Set

4. Myofibrillar Hypertrophy Sets

5. Sarcoplasmic Hypertrophy Sets

Let's go over each.

WARM-UP SETS

The purpose of the warm-up is to infuse enough blood into the muscle and connective tissues so that they can be maximally recruited to handle the heavy sets that follow.

A proper warm-up is an important part of any routine: it helps prevent injury and increases strength.

The warm-up routine I recommend for *Beyond Bigger Leaner Stronger* is simply the warm-up routine found in *BLS*. It's simple and works, so why change it?

Here's how it goes:

First Set:

In your first warm-up set, you want to do 12 reps with about 50% of the weight you normally use for your Myofibrillar Hypertrophy Sets, and then you rest for 1 minute. Don't rush this set, but don't take it too slowly either. It will feel very light and easy.

So, if you did 3 sets of 5 with 275 on the bench last week, you would start your warm-up at 135 and do 12 reps, followed by 1 minute of rest.

Second Set:

In your second set, you use the same weight as the first and do 10 reps, this time at a little faster pace. Then rest for 1 minute.

Third Set:

Your third set is 4 reps with about 70% of the weight you normally use for your Myofibrillar Hypertrophy Sets, and you should do it at a moderate pace. It should still feel light and easy. This set and the following one are to acclimate your muscles to the heavy weights that are about to come. Once again, you follow this with a 1-minute rest.

With a Myofibrillar Hypertrophy Set weight of 275, this would be about 190 to 195 pounds.

Fourth Set:

The fourth set is the final warm-up set, and it's very simple: one rep with about 90% of your Myofibrillar Hypertrophy Set weight. This is to fully acclimate your muscles to the heavy sets that you're about to start. Then rest 2 to 3 minutes before starting your next set.

This would be about 250 pounds if your heavy weight is 275.

Once you've completed these 4 sets, you're ready to begin your heavy lifting (your working sets), starting with Power Sets.

POWER SETS

For all workouts but arms, you will start your workouts with Power Sets, which are for pure strength training. (We'll talk about the difference for arms soon.)

This will entail working with heavy weights that allow for no more than 2 to 3 reps (90%+ of your 1RM), and you will always be doing compound exercises like the Squat, Deadlift, Bench Press, and Military Press.

Power Sets are short (10 to 15 seconds) and should be performed using a 2–1–1 tempo. This means 2 seconds down (the negative portion of the rep), a slight pause, and an explosive movement upward.

Rest 3 to 5 minutes in between each Power Set.

ONE-REP MAX SETS

The One-Rep Max Set is a part of your Power Week, and it involves using the amount of weight that you can only perform one rep with.

Generally speaking, it's about 10 pounds more than the weight you use for your Power Sets. For example, if you can Squat 405 for 2, then your 1RM will be about 415.

One-Rep Max Sets are short (about 5 seconds) and should be performed using a 2–1–1 tempo.

Rest 4 to 5 minutes in between each One-Rep Max Set.

MYOFIBRILLAR HYPERTROPHY SETS

After your power training, you'll move on to sets performed in the 4 to 6 rep range (80% to 85% of your 1RM).

These sets will also focus on compound lifts, although not as purely compound as the Power Sets (for example, your Power Sets on back day will begin with Deadlifts, and your Myofibrillar Sets might begin with Barbell Rows).

Myofibrillar Sets take a little longer to complete (20 to 25 seconds) and should be performed with a 2–1–1 tempo.

Rest 2 to 3 minutes in between each Myofibrillar Set.

SARCOPLASMIC HYPERTROPHY SETS

Last are your Sarcoplasmic Hypertrophy Sets, which entail working in the 8 to 10 rep range (70% to 75% of your 1RM).

These sets will generally involve compound lifting, but some isolation work will be included here.

Sarcoplasmic sets take even longer to complete (30 to 40 seconds) and should be performed with a 3–1–2 tempo.

Rest 1 or 2 minutes in between each Sarcoplasmic Set.

Okay, now that you understand the types of sets you will be doing, let's look at how they factor into the three different types of weeks in the mesocycle.

(Keep in mind the following workouts assume you will be training 5 to 6 times per week. If you will be training 3 to 4 times per week, it's a bit different, which we'll discuss shortly.)

NORMAL WEEK WORKOUT

During a Normal Week, all workouts except those for shoulders and arms will look like this (we'll discuss the differences for shoulders and arms training in a minute):

Warm-up:

2 Power Sets

6 Myofibrillar Hypertrophy Sets

2 Sarcoplasmic Hypertrophy Sets

As you can see, the focus here is myofibrillar muscle growth, and it's supplemented with power and sarcoplasmic training. Calf and ab training will be done addition to the above routine.

Here's an example of a Normal Week chest workout:

Warm-up:

You will do your 4 warm-up sets on the Bench Press, which is where your power training will begin.

Power Sets:

2 x Bench Press

Myofibrillar Sets:

3 x Incline Bench Press

3 x Incline Dumbbell Press

Sarcoplasmic Sets:

2 x Dips (weighted if possible)

Simple enough.

POWER WEEK WORKOUT

For your Power Weeks, you will train all muscle groups except arms like this:

Warm-Up:

2 Power Sets

1 One-Rep Max Set

3 Myofibrillar Hypertrophy Sets

2 Sarcoplasmic Hypertrophy Sets

It's *tough*, but remember that the stronger you get, the more you can get out of your myofibrillar and sarcoplasmic training.

Here's an example of a Power Week back workout:

Warm-up:

You'll do your 4 warm-up sets with the Deadlift, which is where your power training will begin.

Power Sets:

2 x Deadlift

One-Rep Max Set:

1 x Deadlift

Myofibrillar Sets:

3 x Barbell Row

Sarcoplasmic Sets:

2 x Pull-Ups (weighted if possible)

I personally love this workout. The rush of blasting your back with heavy weight is just great fun.

DELOAD OR REST WEEK

Each mesocycle ends with a Deload Week, or a week of complete rest. In case you're not familiar with the term, deloading refers to using much lighter weights than usual to give your body a break while still maintaining strength.

There are two ways I like to deload:

1. Five workouts per week, one major muscle group per workout, 9 sets per workout, compound exercises, and 10 reps with about 40% of 1RM per set, 1 minute rest in between sets. These workouts are easy. You never push to failure or even try to fatigue your muscles much. You're basically just getting a bit of a pump.

2. Three workouts per week, push-pull-legs split, 9 sets per workout, compound lifts, and 10 reps with about 40% of your 1RM per set, 1 minute rest in between sets.

With this deload protocol, your push workout is Bench Press,

Military Press, and Close-Grip Bench Press; your pull workout is Deadlift, Barbell Row, and Pull-Up; and your legs workout is Squat, Barbell Lunge, and Leg Press.

Again, these are easy workouts. You don't go to failure or fatigue: you get a pump and leave.

As it sounds, a Rest Week means a week completely off the weights. This can be necessary depending on how overloaded your system is by the end of the mesocycle.

Personally, I prefer a Deload Week and have been leaning toward the 3-day routine as of late and have been liking it. Some people do better with a Rest Week though. This is one of those things you just play by how you're feeling.

AN IMPORTANT POINT ON REP RANGES

This may not need to be said, but it's an important point, so bear with me.

When I talk about working in a given rep range, what I mean is using an amount of weight that allows for at least the low number but no more than the high number.

For example, the 4 to 6 rep range calls for an amount of weight that allows at least 4 but no more than 6 reps.

If you're wondering what you're supposed to do once you hit the upper end of a given rep range, we'll go over that soon.

So, that's what you will be doing in your workouts. The next piece of the puzzle is training frequency. How often will you be doing these workouts, and why?

TRAINING FREQUENCY IN BEYOND BIGGER LEANER STRONGER

Optimal training frequency is a hotly debated subject.

Some people believe that you must train your entire body 2 to 3 times per week to make gains, whereas others believe that such an approach will only lead to overtraining.

Further complicating the matter is the fact that people have made all kinds of crazy training routines "work" in terms of building muscle and strength. Recommendations run the gamut from extremely low workout volumes (1 or 2 sets per muscle group) repeated several times per week to extremely high volumes (20 to 25 sets per muscle group) done more infrequently. In many cases, the people who make gains with such approaches are on drugs.

The truth is optimal training frequency as a natural weightlifter depends on what you're doing in each workout, both in terms of volume and intensity.

Finding scientific help on the matter of optimal training volume is tough due to the number of variables involved, but something of an answer can be found in a large review conducted by researchers at Goteborg University.[18]

I'll get straight to the point and quote the research: "Overall, moderate volumes (~30 to 60 repetitions per session for [Dynamic External Resistance] training) appear to yield the largest responses."

This range has a lot of anecdotal support and is commonly recommended by educated, experienced weightlifters and bodybuilders. If you look at many of the popular, tried-and-true routines out there, the workout volume generally falls in there somewhere.

For example, my *BLS* program has you do 9 to 12 sets of 4 to 6 reps per major muscle group. You move up in weight once you get 6 reps (which usually knocks your next set down to 4 reps), so the workouts range between 45 and 60 high-intensity reps. And people make fantastic strength and size gains on the program.

The program in this book also has you doing about 60 reps per workout, with a combination of very high-intensity, high-intensity, and moderate-intensity work. This workout volume—both the number of reps and the intensities used—has both scientific and anecdotal evidence on its side. It works, period.

So, if that's the workout volume, let's get back to the matter of training frequency.

In *BLS*, I recommend people lift weights 5 times per week and take 2 days off weightlifting. Each body part gets its own day (chest, back, shoulders, arms, legs), and thus each body part gets directly trained once per week.

Some people believe that such an approach is doomed—that each muscle group needs at least two full workouts per week to grow bigger and stronger. Both anecdotal evidence and clinical research says otherwise, though.

I have scores of success stories on my website to prove that training each major muscle group once per 5 to 7 days produces phenomenal results, and research shows that proper workout volume and intensity appear to be more important than frequency.[19] [20]

The bad rap that "one-muscle-group-per-day" splits get is mainly due to poor program design: poor exercise choice, rep range emphasis, and workout volume. Most one-a-day splits involve too much isolation work with low weight for high reps, which results in low workout intensity with volumes that are far too high.

"But what about protein synthesis rates?" you might be thinking. "Aren't muscles fully recovered in 2 to 3 days, ready to get hit again?"

Well, research has shown that muscle protein synthesis rates spike at about 24 hours after a workout and return to normal by about 36 hours.[21] This means that theoretically you should train each muscle group once every 2 to 3 days to stimulate maximum muscle growth, and there are weightlifting programs built around this principle.

These programs can work, but a common problem people run into with them is related to recovery. As training volume and intensity increases, so does the amount of time it takes for your muscles to fully recover, as measured by performance capacity.

Research has shown that even in resistance-trained, college-aged men, full muscle recovery can take anywhere from 48 to 96 hours depending on how they trained, ate, and slept, as well as other physiological factors like hormones and genetics.[22] If we look at other recovery-related studies, we see that most people's muscles take closer to 72 – 96 hours to fully recover from an intense weightlifting session, that older men need more time to recover than young, and that larger muscles need more time to recover than smaller.[23]

Furthermore, muscular recovery is only part of the picture. Intense weightlifting places a lot of stress on the nervous system, and research has shown that this fatigue can "accumulate" from workout to workout.[24] If it becomes too great, overtraining symptoms set in, which includes a dramatic reduction in performance, depression, sleep disturbances, and more.

This is why I made to switch from erring on the side of training too frequently to ensuring each muscle group gets enough rest between each workout. It's also worth noting that by focusing on compound lifts in each workout, you actually are training more than just the day's muscle group. For instance, the Deadlift and Squat trains a lot more than just your back and legs.

The bottom line is the combination of proper training volume and high workout intensity using a once-per-week split works incredibly well with *BLS*, and it's equally effective with *Beyond Bigger Leaner Stronger*.

That is, the recommended approach to the *Beyond Bigger Leaner Stronger* program is to lift weights 5 or 6 days per week, focusing on one or two major muscle groups per day, with 1 or 2 days of rest (no weightlifting, but cardio is allowed).

Here's a very standard Monday to Friday approach (my preferred approach):

Day 1:
Chest & Abs

Day 2:
Back & Calves

Day 3:
Shoulders

Day 4:
Arms & Abs

Day 5:
Legs

Day 6:
Cardio or Rest

Day 7:
Cardio or Rest

Rest days can be interspersed, however:

Day 1:

Chest & Abs

Day 2:

Back & Calves

Day 3:

Rest

Day 4:

Arms & Abs

Day 5:

Shoulders

Day 6:

Legs

Day 7:

Rest

The order of muscle groups trained can be tweaked as well:

Day 1:

Legs

Day 2:

Chest & Abs

Day 3:

Arms

Day 4:

Back & Calves

Day 5:

Shoulders & Abs

Day 6:

Cardio

Day 7:

Rest

If weak point training were included (we'll talk about this more soon), it might look like this:

Day 1:

Chest & Abs

Day 2:

Back & Calves

Day 3:

Shoulders

Day 4:

Arms & Abs

Day 5:

Legs

Day 6:

Shoulders & Back (weak points)

Day 7:

Rest

So, that's the basic layout of your week. You can play with training and rest days and work them around your schedule and preferences.

THE CORE EXERCISES OF THE BEYOND BIGGER LEANER STRONGER PROGRAM

A big part of what makes this program effective is the exercises performed.

As you would expect, the majority of your lifting will be done with compound, free-weight exercises, as these are just the most effective for building strength and size. There is a place for isolation movements, and you will be doing some, but they should never be the emphasis of a workout.

Let's go through the exercises that you should use to program your workouts, and then we'll go over some basic workout programming theory.

CHEST

For your Power Sets, you should choose from the following exercises:

Incline Barbell Bench Press
Flat Barbell Bench Press
Incline Dumbbell Press
Flat Dumbbell Press

That's it. Those are the staple exercises for building a big and strong chest, and they are all great choices for your Power Sets.

For your Myofibrillar Sets, you should choose from the following exercises:

Incline Barbell Bench Press
Flat Barbell Bench Press
Incline Dumbbell Press
Flat Dumbbell Press
Weighted Dip

Because you're still handling heavy weights here and pushing for myofibrillar hypertrophy, you stick to the same mass-building exercises as your Power Sets, with the additional option of Weighted Dips.

For your Sarcoplasmic Sets, you should choose from the following exercises:

Incline Barbell Bench Press
Flat Barbell Bench Press
Incline Dumbbell Press
Flat Dumbbell Press
Weighted Dips
Dumbbell Fly (Incline and Flat)

The only addition here is the dumbbell fly, which doesn't work so well in the 4 to 6 rep range (it's quite hard on the shoulders) but is effective in the 8 to 10 rep range.

BACK

For your Power Sets, you should choose from the following exercises:

Barbell Deadlift

Barbell Row

The most important lift out of these two is the Deadlift, and it should be included in every back workout, whether as Power or Myofibrillar Sets or both.

For your Myofibrillar Sets, you should choose from the following exercises:

Barbell Deadlift

Barbell Row

T-Bar Row

One-Arm Dumbbell Row

Pull-Up (weighted if possible)

Front-Lat Pulldown (Wide-Grip and Close-Grip)

V-Bar Pulldown

These are the best mass-builders for your back and are all you need for your myofibrillar training.

For your Sarcoplasmic Sets, you should choose from the following exercises:

Barbell Row

T-Bar Row (Barbell or Machine)

One-Arm Dumbbell Row

Pull-Up (weighted if possible)

Front-Lat Pulldown (Wide-Grip and Close-Grip)

V-Bar Pulldown

Seated Cable Row

As you can see, a bit of the isolation work fits in here.

SHOULDERS

For your Power Sets, you should choose from the following exercises:

Seated Military Press
Seated Dumbbell Press

Your Power Sets are limited to these two exercises because they're the only three that can be safely done with that much weight.

Note that for your Power Sets, the Seated Military Press is best performed in a Military Press station or in a power cage with a utility bench. Do NOT try performing Power Sets standing or sitting on a flat bench.

For your Myofibrillar Sets, you should choose from the following exercises:

Military Press (Seated or Standing)
Seated Dumbbell Press
Arnold Press
Dumbbell Side Lateral Raise
Dumbbell Front Raise
Barbell Shrugs

Side lateral raises can be particularly hard in this rep range, even if you have the shoulder strength. Something that helps me overcome the issue is to perform them as Leaning Side Raises. To see how these are done, just check out the bonus report at the end of the book—it has a link to a video showing you proper form.

For your Sarcoplasmic Sets, you should choose from the following exercises:

Dumbbell Side Lateral Raise
Dumbbell Front Raise
Dumbbell Rear Dealt Raise (Seated or Bent-Over)
Barbell Rear Delt Row

The sarcoplasmic range is great for your isolation exercises and for targeting the smaller side and rear delts.

LEGS

For your Power Sets, you should choose from the following exercises:

Barbell Back Squat

Barbell Front Squat

Your leg workouts should always start with one of these. There's just no better way to build leg size and strength.

For your Myofibrillar Sets, you should choose from the following exercises:

Barbell Back Squat
Barbell Front Squat
Leg Press
Hack Squat (plate-loaded sled, not barbell)
Romanian Deadlift

As expected, we're sticking with the big compound lifts for the Myofibrillar Sets.

For your Sarcoplasmic Sets, you should choose from the following exercises:

Barbell Back Squat
Barbell Front Squat
Leg Press
Hack Squat (plate-loaded sled, not barbell)
Romanian Deadlift
Barbell Lunge
Dumbbell Lunge
Leg Extension
Leg Curl

Here we have the addition of some lunges and machines, which become viable in this rep range. As a sidenote, leg extensions and curls are always paired with each other or with another exercise that targets the other part of the leg (extensions, which target the quads, can be paired with Romanian Deadlifts, which target the hamstrings, for instance).

Calves seem to respond best to a combination of myofibrillar and sarcoplasmic training. The exercises used are short and simple:

Seated Calf Raise
Standing Calf Raise

Calf Press on the Leg Press

If your calves are already big enough, you don't have to train them directly (they do get trained when you do Deadlifts and Squats).

However, if you want to gain some size, then I recommend you train them 2 to 3 times per week, with 6 to 9 sets per workout.

You can do the same exercises in these workouts, but you want to alternate between focusing exclusively on myofibrillar growth in one workout and sarcoplasmic in the next. That is, in one workout, all sets are in the 4 to 6 rep range. In the next, the 8 to 10 range. If you're training them a third time in the week, it goes back to myofibrillar, and so forth.

To save time, I like to work my calf sets in while I'm resting the major muscle group being trained. I make sure to get at least 60 seconds of rest after the calf set (before performing my next major muscle group set) to bring my heart rate down.

ARMS

There aren't any Power Sets for arms because it just isn't very feasible. The best you could is the Barbell Curl for biceps and Close-Grip Bench Press for triceps, but arms seem to respond best to just myofibrillar and sarcoplasmic training.

For your biceps Myofibrillar Sets, you should choose from the following exercises:

Barbell Curl

E-Z Bar Curl

Dumbbell Curl

Hammer Curl

These are the core exercises for building your biceps. No cable or machine work.

For your triceps Myofibrillar Sets, you should choose from the following exercises:

Close-Grip Bench Press

Seated Triceps Press

Lying Triceps Extension

Weighted Dip (Triceps Version)

My favorites out of these are the Close-Grip Bench Press and Seated Triceps Press, but I will rotate that pair with the Lying Triceps Extension and Weighted Dip.

For your biceps Sarcoplasmic Sets, you should choose from the following exercises:

Barbell Curl

E-Z Bar Curl

Dumbbell Curl

Hammer Curl

Nothing changes here. There's just no reason to move to machines or cables when you can stick to the free weights.

For your triceps Sarcoplasmic Sets, you should choose from the following exercises:

Close-Grip Bench Press

Seated Triceps Press

Lying Triceps Press

Weighted Dip (Triceps Version)

Triceps Pushdown

Here we see the addition of the Triceps Pushdown, which seems to work best in this range.

ABS

Abs are always trained with Sarcoplasmic Sets or with no weight at all. My two favorite ways of training them are as follows:

1. Do 3 to 4 sets of a weighted exercise in the 8 to 10 rep range, 4 times per week.

2. An abs circuit consisting of 3 exercised performed in a row (supetsets), without rest. The circuit looks like this: one weighted set (8 to 10 rep range), followed immediately by a weighted (8 to 10 rep range) or unweighted set to failure, followed immediately by another weighted or unweighted set to failure.

For instance, it could look like this:

1. *Weighted Cable Crunch*

2. *Captain's Chair Leg Raise (with straight legs)*

3. *Air Bicycles*

Or like this:

1. *Hanging Leg Raise (weighted by snatching a dumbbell in between your feet)*

2. *Captain's Chair Leg Raise (with straight legs)*

3. *Air Bicycles*

These exercises are always done back-to-back (supersets), followed by 60 – 90 seconds of rest. 3 to 4 of these circuits would comprise the whole abs workout. I'll let you decide how you want to train your abs and on which days to work them in.

In terms of working these ab circuits into your other workouts, I recommend you complete your major muscle group and do your abs circuits last, which only adds about 7 minutes to your workout.

FINDING YOUR WEIGHTS FOR THE PROGRAM

You can go about finding your weights for the program two ways:

1. Trial and error, using your first 1 or 2 weeks to dial everything in

2. Calculating your 1RMs and using these calculations to predict where your weights will be for each rep range you'll be working in

Both work just fine.

If you're going to use the first method, a rule of thumb that helps is that for every 10 pounds you add to a barbell exercise, you generally lose 2 reps, and the same goes for moving up 5 pounds on your dumbbell exercises.

For instance, if you can bench press 250 pounds for 8 reps, you will probably get 6 reps at 260. If you're pressing 115-pound dumbbells for 8 reps, you'll probably get 6 reps with 120-pound dumbbells.

To find your 1RM for a given lift, use an amount of weight that allows for about 4 to 6 reps, and use the following equation:

Weight x Reps x 0.0333 + Weight = Estimated 1RM

For example, if I can squat 335 for 5 reps, then the equation looks like this:

(335 x 5) 1,675 x 0.0333 = 56 + 335 = 391

What you will want to do is look over the exercises that you will be performing in the next mesocycle of the program and use your most recent performance of those exercises to calculate your 1RMs.

Then, take those 1RMs and modify them as follows to guesstimate the weights you will use for your mesocycle:

Power Sets:
90% of your 1RM

Myofibrillar Sets:
80% of your 1RM

Sarcoplasmic Sets:
70% of your 1RM

Remember that these calculations are estimates, and depending on your level of conditioning, they may or may not hold true for you.

If you find you can do more than 3 reps with 90% of your 1RM as calculated earlier, then just add weight for your next set. If you find you can only get 1 rep or none, don't be dismayed—simply lower the weight for your next set and carry on.

The same goes for each of the other rep ranges. Increase or decrease weights as needed to figure out exactly where you're at.

PROGRESSING ON THE PROGRAM

As with *BLS*, your primary goal in this program is to continue adding weight to the bar over time.

You do this by increasing weight by once you hit the top end of the rep range you're working in. Specifically, you increase by 5 total pounds for One-Rep Max and Power Sets, and by 10 total pounds for Myofibrillar and Sarcoplasmic Sets.

For example, if you're doing your first Power Set of Squats and get

3 reps, add 5 pounds for your second set (2.5 pounds to each side of the bar), and you should be able to get 2 reps on your next set. If you're doing a Power Set with dumbbells, then you move up to the next set (a 5-pound increase in each dumbbell).

The same goes for all other sets: when you hit 6 reps with a given weight in your myofibrillar training, go up by 10 pounds (5 pounds added to each side of the bar, or a 5-pound increase in each dumbbell). When you hit 10 reps in your sarcoplasmic training, go up in the same way.

By doing this, you'll ensure you're always increasing tension in the muscle fibers and keeping them progressively overloaded.

If you hit the top of your rep range, move up in weight, and then do less reps than the bottom of your rep range on the next set, move back to the original weight and work with it until you can hit the top of your rep range for two sets in a row. You then try to move up again and see if you can at least get enough reps to hit the bottom of your rep range.

For example, let's say you're performing your first Myofibrillar Set and get 6 reps. You move up in weight and then only get 3 reps on the next set. You should move back to the original 6-rep weight and work with that until you can get two sets of 6 reps with it, and then try to move up again. You should then be able to get 4 reps with the new, higher weight.

If, even after working until you can get two 6-rep sets, you still couldn't get 4 reps with the higher weight, you can work with the original weight until you can get three 6-rep sets, and then you will almost certainly be able to move up properly.

Now, it may happen that you go up in your power training and then have trouble with the weights you were using during last week's myofibrillar training, or go up in your myofibrillar training and then struggle with your sarcoplasmic training, and that's okay. It can happen (your muscles are a little extra fatigued from the weight increase). Just reduce the weight for your remaining sets to keep you in the proper rep range, and your performance in all rep ranges will increase over time.

TRAINING YOUR SHOULDERS AND ARMS

As you know, shoulders and arms are trained a bit differently than other muscle groups. Let's look at shoulders first.

SHOULDERS TRAINING

A Normal Week shoulders workout can and should follow the normal pattern laid out earlier, but some people find it necessary to work in the 6 to 8 or the 8 to 10 rep range for the Side and Front Lateral Raise. While they have no issues with heavy presses, they simply can't maintain proper form with heavy weight on these exercises.

If that happens, then just work in a higher rep range and, as you get stronger, try to move back into the 4 to 6 rep range.

ARMS TRAINING

The major difference with arms training is there are no Power Sets whatsoever. Two- and One-Rep Max Sets just aren't feasible with arms training—form goes to hell and joints get achy, fast.

Instead, your arms workouts for both Normal and Power Weeks should look like this for both biceps and triceps:

4 Myofibrillar Hypertrophy Sets

2 Sarcoplasmic Hypertrophy Sets

That is, you'll be doing 4 Myofibrillar Hypertrophy Sets followed by 2 Sarcoplasmic Hypertrophy Sets for both biceps and triceps, for a total workout volume of 12 sets.

When I'm warming up my arms, I like to superset the sets to get it done quicker (biceps warm-up set, directly into triceps warm-up set, rest 60 seconds, repeat until warm-up is complete).

Once I've begun the heavy lifting, I like to work my arms like this:

Biceps exercise 1 set 1

Rest 60 to 90 seconds

Triceps exercise 1 set 1

Rest 60 to 90 seconds

Biceps exercise 1 set 2

Rest 60 to 90 seconds

Triceps exercise 1 set 2
Rest 60 to 90 seconds

And so forth. This lets me finish my workout in 45 minutes or so. Some people prefer to train biceps or triceps first, with rest times as laid out earlier, and then train the other. This takes a bit longer but is fine as well.

IF YOU CAN'T TRAIN 5 OR 6 TIMES PER WEEK

Work, family, other obligations…I understand.

If you can't fit in 5 or 6 lifting days per week, you can still do the program if you can train at least 3 times per week (and 4 is even better, of course).

FOUR TRAINING DAYS PER WEEK

If you can only train 4 days per week, the solution is simple. You can follow the 5-day workout plans I give in this book and in the bonus report, but you modify them in one of two ways:

1. Drop arms day if you don't feel they need to grow anymore. It's common for guys to be happy with their arm size after 2 to 3 years of lifting. If that's you, you can drop that day, and your back, chest, and shoulders days will hit your arms enough to maintain their size and strength.

2. Combine muscle groups. The muscle groups to merge into other days are shoulders or arms. For instance, you can do chest and triceps together and back and biceps together, or you can move shoulders to legs day. (I prefer the former.)

Here are a few tips for making this work:

CHEST AND TRICEPS AND BACK AND BICEPS

If you're going to go this route, then I recommend reducing the normal workout volume for your arms. Drop to 2 Myofibrillar Hypertrophy Sets and 2 Sarcoplasmic for both biceps and triceps, or just 4 Myofibrillar Hypertrophy Sets for each.

You can do these sets after you finish your chest workout, or you can begin them when you get to your Sarcoplasmic Hypertrophy Sets for chest and back. What I like to do is my chest/back set, rest 60 to 90 seconds, arms set, rest 60 to 90 seconds, chest/back set, rest 60 to 90 seconds, arms set, etc. For example:

Chest exercise 1 set 1

Rest 60 to 90 seconds

Triceps exercise 1 set 1

Rest 60 to 90 seconds

Chest exercise 1 set 2

Rest 60 to 90 seconds

Triceps exercise 1 set 2

Rest 60 to 90 seconds

You should use the normal warm-up routine for your chest, but you won't need to warm up your arms.

LEGS AND SHOULDERS

I'm not going to lie—this is a *tough* workout. But some people prefer it over the above option.

To make this work, train your legs first, followed by your shoulders. I don't recommend reducing the workout volume of either. If you're tight on your rest times, you should be able to finish it all in about 1:15 to 1:30, which isn't too bad.

Fully warm up each muscle group.

Now, in case you're worried that combining workouts like this will lead to overtraining due to the number of reps per workout far exceeding the recommend limits, remember that our discussion earlier applied to muscle groups trained per workout, not to the entire workout itself.

That is, *each muscle group* should receive around 60 reps of training per workout, but the overall workout can contain more than 60 reps.

For your Deload Week, you can simply follow the 3-day protocol given earlier.

THREE TRAINING DAYS PER WEEK

If you can only train three days per week, then you will follow what is known as a push-pull-legs split. As it sounds, it has you train your "push" muscles on day 1 (chest, shoulders, and triceps), your "pull" muscles on day 2 (back and biceps), and your legs on day three.

First, let's clarify the warm-up routine on the three-day split.

- For your push day, you should do a full warm-up routine for both your chest and shoulders. I like to first warm up my chest and perform my chest Power Sets and then warm up my shoulders and perform their Power Sets.

- For your pull day, you should do a full warm-up on your back, but no warm-up is needed for biceps.

- For your legs day, you should do a full warm-up.

Your three-day Normal Week workout will look like this:

2 or 4 Power Sets

6 Myofibrillar Hypertrophy Sets

2 to 4 Sarcoplasmic Hypertrophy Sets

Here's an example:

Day 1: Push

Warm up chest
Power Sets:
2 x Incline Barbell Bench Press
2 x Military Press or Overhead Press
Myofibrillar Sets:
3 x Flat Barbell Bench Press
3 x Dumbbell Shoulder Press
Sarcoplasmic Sets:
2 x Dips (weighted if possible)
2 x Close-Grip Bench Press

Day 2: Pull

Warm up
Power Sets:
2 x Deadlift
Myofibrillar Sets:
3 x Barbell Row

3 x One-Arm Dumbbell Row
Sarcoplasmic Sets:
2 x Pull-ups (weighted if possible)
2 x Barbell Curl

Day 3: Legs

Warm up
Power Sets:
2 x Barbell Squat
Myofibrillar Sets:
3 x Romanian Deadlift
3 x Hack Squat (sled, not barbell) or Barbell Lunge (Walking or In-Place) if no sled
3 x Calf Press on the Leg Press
Sarcoplasmic Sets:
2 x Leg Press
2 x Standing Calf Raise

Fairly simple.

Your three-day Power Week will look like this:

2 Power Sets
1 or 2 One-Rep Max Sets
4 Myofibrillar Hypertrophy Sets
2 or 4 Sarcoplasmic Hypertrophy Sets

And here's how to lay these sets out:

Day 1: Push

Warm up chest
Power Sets:
1 x Incline Barbell Bench Press
One-Rep Max Sets:
1 x Incline Barbell Bench Press
Power Sets:
1 x Military Press or Overhead Press

One-Rep Max Sets:
1 x Military Press or Overhead Press
Myofibrillar Sets:
2 x Flat Barbell Bench Press
2 x Dumbbell Shoulder Press
Sarcoplasmic Sets:
2 x Dips (Chest Version, weighted if possible)
2 x Close-Grip Bench Press

As you can see, the Power and One-Rep Max Sets are separated by exercise for the sake of convenience. You would warm up your chest, do your first Power Set, add weight and rest, do your One-Rep Max Set, and then move on to your Military Presses. You shouldn't have to do any additional warm-up work for your shoulders.

Day 2: Pull

Warm up
Power Sets:
2 x Deadlift
One-Rep Max Set:
1 x Deadlift
Myofibrillar Sets:
2 x Barbell Row
2 x One-Arm Dumbbell Row
Sarcoplasmic Sets:
2 x Pull-ups (weighted if possible)
2 x Barbell Curl

Day 3: Legs

Warm up

Power Sets:
2 x Barbell Squat
One-Rep Max Set:
1 x Barbell Squat

Myofibrillar Sets:
2 x Romanian Deadlift
2 x Hack Squat or Barbell Lunge
Sarcoplasmic Sets:
2 x Leg Press
2 x Calf Press on the Leg Press
2 x Standing Calf Raise

For your Deload Week, you can simply follow the 3-day protocol given earlier.

Okay, you now understand the overall layout of the program and what types of workouts you're supposed to do and when.

Let's now explore the practical details of doing the workouts and progressing through the program.

WHEN TO CHANGE EXERCISES IN YOUR ROUTINE

As you'll see in the sample workouts following this section, you will be doing the same exercises throughout each mesocycle. You will not be changing your workouts every week.

The reason for this is you don't gain anything by changing exercises frequently. In fact, you can set yourself back because by the time you feel grooved in with an exercise in terms of form and proper weight, you're changing it to something else. It also makes it hard to know if you're progressing, because you can't see if you're moving up in weight on certain exercises over time.

The only good reason to change to another exercise in the middle of a mesocycle is trouble like achy joints, muscle strains, etc.

So, when it comes time to program your own routine, I recommend you follow this principle: if you want to switch exercises, do it before starting a new mesocycle.

How often you should change exercises will depend a lot on how your body responds to training. If you're making great gains on your mesocycle and want to continue it longer than 6 weeks, then you're free to do so.

On the flip side, if you're really not liking a particular exercise, don't be afraid to change it out before starting a new mesocycle. Different bodies respond differently to exercises, and you learn your body by trying different things.

HOW TO MODIFY THE PROGRAM DUE TO AGE

If you're an advanced weightlifter but aren't sure if you can do the program due to your age, I have simple advice for you.

The first point relates to heavy bench pressing, military pressing, squatting, and deadlifting. These exercises aren't inherently dangerous, but if you've sustained joint injuries in the past or have other structural weaknesses, it's best to avoid the 1 to 3 rep range on these lifts.

Instead, you can modify the program as follows:

1. For your Normal Weeks, replace the Power Sets with Myofibrillar Hypertrophy Sets or with one Myofibrillar Set and one Sarcoplasmic Hypertrophy Set (but keep the order in which you perform them—Myofibrillar Sets first, followed by Sarcoplasmic Sets).

2. Drop Power Weeks and follow Normal Weeks only.

Another point is to simply listen to your body. If you feel the symptoms of overtraining setting in after 4 weeks, then take your Deload Week early. Remember that recovery is key.

All right. That wraps up the nuts and bolts of the program. If you're feeling overwhelmed, I understand—it's a lot to take in. Check out the next chapter, which has recommended workouts for your first mesocycle, and feel free to then come back and reread this chapter to make sure everything is clear.

WHAT TO DO
IF YOU BEGIN FEELING OVERTRAINED

This program is deceptively tough. Ten sets in a workout doesn't seem like anything particularly grueling, but the emphasis on heavy compound lifting takes a lot out of you.

You shouldn't have any trouble doing the program so long as you take your Rest and Deload Weeks, but you may run into signs of overtraining (general fatigue, sleep problems, decrease in strength, unusual aches and pains, depression, and so forth).

If this happens, the first thing you should do is ensure your diet is right, you're getting enough sleep, and you're not doing too much exercise in addition to your weightlifting. Eating too little food and/or too little protein is a surefire way to become overtrained, getting too little sleep is even worse, and too much cardio or other exercise will over-stress the body.

If you're feeling overtrained despite eating right, getting plenty of sleep, and not over-exercising, don't fret. It can happen. This program puts a lot of stress on the body and sometimes you just need to dial it back a bit. There are two ways I like to do this:

1. Replace one Normal Week with *BLS* workouts, so each mesocycle looks like this:

   1 *BLS* Week

   3 Normal Weeks

   1 Power Week

   1 Rest or Deload Week

2. Remove one Normal Week from your mesocycles, making each mesocycle look like this:

   3 Normal Weeks

   1 Power Week

   1 Rest or Deload Week

I prefer the first remedy, but both work well.

After one modified mesocycle, see how your body feels. If the overtraining symptoms are gone, you can go back to the normal routine. If you still feel less than 100%, continue with another modified mesocycle and you should be up to snuff.

8

YOUR FIRST *BEYOND BIGGER LEANER STRONGER* WORKOUTS

WHILE YOU'RE MORE THAN WELCOME TO start creating your own routine using the exercises and principles discussed thus far, I want to make sure you have no issues getting started on the program.

So in the following pages I'm going to lay out the workouts for the first mesocycle of the program. And as mentioned earlier, you can find a full year's worth of workouts in the bonus report, which you can access through the link provided at the end of the book.

Keep in mind that the order in which you train your muscles can be adapted to suit your preferences or schedule. I prefer the following order because it gives everything enough rest before getting hit again, but there are other ways to arrange the days and accomplish the same.

Let's look at the workouts for the first mesocycle of the 5-day split first. And remember, you decide where you want to insert your ab training.

5-DAY SPLIT PHASE 1:
NORMAL WEEK:

DAY 1: CHEST

Warm-Up

Power Sets:
2 x Incline Barbell Bench Press

Myofibrillar Sets:
3 x Incline Dumbbell Press
3 x Flat Barbell Bench Press

Sarcoplasmic Sets:
2 x Dips (weighted if possible)

DAY 2: BACK & CALVES

Warm-Up

Power Sets:
2 x Deadlift

Myofibrillar Sets:
2 x Deadlift
2 x Barbell Row
2 x One-Arm Dumbbell Row
3 x Calf Press on the Leg Press
3 x Standing Calf Raise

Sarcoplasmic Sets:
2 x Pull-Ups (weighted if possible)

DAY 3: SHOULDERS

Warm-Up
Power Sets:
2 x Military Press or Overhead Press

Myofibrillar Sets:
3 x Dumbbell Shoulder Press
3 x Dumbbell Side Lateral Raise

Sarcoplasmic Sets:
2 x Seated or Bent-Over Rear Lateral Raise

DAY 4: ARMS

Warm up both biceps and triceps

Myofibrillar Sets:
2 x Barbell Curl
2 x Close-Grip Bench Press
2 x Dumbbell Curl
2 x Seated Triceps Press

Sarcoplasmic Sets:
2 x Hammer Curl
2 x Triceps Pushdown

DAY 5: LEGS

Warm-Up

Power Sets:
2 x Barbell Squat

Myofibrillar Sets:
2 x Barbell Squat
2 x Romanian Deadlift
2 x Hack Squat or Barbell Lunge

Sarcoplasmic Sets:
2 x Leg Press
3 x Calf Press on the Leg Press
3 x Standing Calf Raise

POWER WEEK:

DAY 1: CHEST

Warm-Up

Power Sets:
2 x Incline Barbell Bench Press

One-Rep Max Set:
1 x Flat Barbell Bench Press

Myofibrillar Sets:
3 x Dips (weighted if possible)

Sarcoplasmic Sets:
2 x Dips (weighted if possible)

DAY 2: BACK

Warm-Up

Power Sets:
2 x Deadlift

One-Rep Max Sets:
1 x Deadlift

Myofibrillar Sets:
3 x Barbell Row

Sarcoplasmic Sets:
2 x Pull-Ups (weighted if possible)

DAY 3: SHOULDERS

Warm-Up

Power Sets:
2 x Military Press or Overhead Press

One-Rep Max Set:
1 x Military Press or Overhead Press

Myofibrillar Sets:
3 x Dumbbell Shoulder Press

Sarcoplasmic Sets:
2 x Dumbbell Side Lateral Raise

DAY 4: ARMS

Warm up both biceps and triceps

Myofibrillar Sets:

2 x Barbell Curl

2 x Close-Grip Bench Press

2 x Dumbbell Curl

2 x Seated Triceps Press

Sarcoplasmic Sets:

2 x Hammer Curl

2 x Triceps Pushdown

DAY 5: LEGS

Warm-Up

Power Sets:

2 x Barbell Squat

One-Rep Max Sets:

1 x Barbell Squat

Myofibrillar Sets:

3 x Romanian Deadlift

3 x Calf Press on the Leg Press

Sarcoplasmic Sets:

2 x Leg Press

3 x Standing Calf Raise

As you know, this phase would then end with a Rest or Deload Week, after which you would begin the second mesocycle (which you can find in the bonus report, or you can program your own).

And in case you're wondering, you do the exercises in the order given (from top to bottom), and you complete one exercise before moving onto the next.

4-DAY SPLIT PHASE 1:

If you're training 4 days per week, you simply adjust the above as discussed earlier (drop arms day or combine muscle groups).

3-DAY SPLIT PHASE 1:

If you're training 3 days per week, you should rest 1 day in between each workout. Many people like to do Monday – Wednesday – Friday.

Here are your Phase 1 workouts:

NORMAL WEEK:

DAY 1: PUSH

Warm up chest
Power Sets:
2 x Incline Barbell Bench Press
Warm up shoulders
Power Sets:
2 x Military Press
Myofibrillar Sets:
3 x Flat Barbell Bench Press
3 x Dumbbell Shoulder Press
Sarcoplasmic Sets:
2 x Dips (weighted if possible)
2 x Close-Grip Bench Press

DAY 2: PULL

Warm-Up
Power Sets:
2 x Deadlift
Myofibrillar Sets:
2 x Deadlift
2 x Barbell Row
2 x One-Arm Dumbbell Row
Sarcoplasmic Sets:
2 x Pull-Ups (weighted if possible)
2 x Barbell Curl

DAY 3: LEGS

Warm-Up
Power Sets:
2 x Barbell Squat
Myofibrillar Sets:

2 x Barbell Squat
2 x Romanian Deadlift
2 x Hack Squat or Barbell Lunge
Sarcoplasmic Sets:
2 x Leg Press
3 x Calf Press on the Leg Press
3 x Standing Calf Raise

POWER WEEK:

DAY 1: PUSH

Warm up chest
Power Sets:
1 x Incline Barbell Bench Press
One-Rep Max Sets:
1 x Incline Barbell Bench Press
Warm up shoulders
Power Sets:
1 x Military Press or Overhead Press
One-Rep Max Sets:
1 x Military Press or Overhead Press
Myofibrillar Sets:
2 x Flat Barbell Bench Press
2 x Dumbbell Shoulder Press
Sarcoplasmic Sets:
2 x Dips (Chest Version, weighted if possible)
2 x Close-Grip Bench Press

DAY 2: PULL

Warm up
Power Sets:
2 x Deadlift
One-Rep Max Set:
1 x Deadlift
Myofibrillar Sets:

2 x Barbell Row

2 x One-Arm Dumbbell Row

Sarcoplasmic Sets:

2 x Pull-ups (weighted if possible)

2 x Barbell Curl

DAY 3: LEGS

Warm up

Power Sets:

2 x Barbell Squat

One-Rep Max Sets:

2 x Barbell Squat

Myofibrillar Sets:

2 x Romanian Deadlift

2 x Hack Squat or Barbell Lunge

Sarcoplasmic Sets:

2 x Leg Press

2 x Calf Press on the Leg Press

2 x Standing Calf Raise

So, while it may seem like a lot to take in at once, that's how the program works, and that's how I recommend you start.

I want to remind you here to make sure you grab the bonus report at the end of book for an entire year's worth of workouts (mesocycles).

In the next chapter, we're going to talk about weak point training and how to properly address the lagging points of your physique with additional training beyond the core workouts laid out so far.

9

HOW TO IMPROVE WEAK POINTS IN YOUR PHYSIQUE

CHANCES ARE YOU FEEL CERTAIN THINGS about your physique are underdeveloped. Or maybe you took your measurements earlier and know for a fact what is behind and what's not.

Many guys complain about their chest and arms being small. For others, like me, it's hard to grow the shoulders fast enough to remain proportionate with the arms.

Genetics are partly to blame for weak points. For example, my chest has always grown quickly, but my shoulders, lats, and calves have always been stubborn. For you, maybe your chest grows slowly but your back or legs explode.

Weak points are usually a result of improper training, however. Many guys simply neglect certain parts of their bodies by focusing on the wrong exercises and by not training them frequently or intensely enough.

Whatever your weak points are, don't worry—you can fix them. And it's very simple to do.

The big "secret" of weak point training is this: you train your weak points more frequently, without going so far as to cause overtraining.

No surprise there. Let's look at the specifics, though, and how you fit weak point training into the *Beyond Bigger Leaner Stronger* program.

HOW WEAK POINT TRAINING WORKS

The key to weak point training is giving the muscle group(s) being targeted enough rest before they are trained again, and not overdoing it in the training.

Specifically, you want to make sure it's been at least 3 to 4 days since you last trained the weak point(s), and you want to perform an additional 2 Myofibrillar and Sarcoplasmic Sets per weak point being addressed.

For example, if you are doing extra chest training, you could do this:

2 Myofibrillar Sets of Incline Bench Press

2 Sarcoplasmic Sets of Flat Bench Press

Or this:

4 Myofibrillar Sets of Weighted Dips

You can do your weak point training in one extra workout per week, on its own day, or you can tack it onto other workouts.

For instance, if you're lifting 5 days per week, you can do your weak point training on the 6th day (and if you're lifting 4 or 3 days per week, you can do your weak point training on the 5th or 4th days, respectively).

Or, if you want to begin or end an existing workout with your weak point training, you can do that as well. For example, if you were doing extra chest training, you could do it like this:

Day 1:

Chest

Day 2:

Back

Day 3:

Shoulders

Day 4:

Arms

Day 5:
Legs & Chest Weak Point Training

Day 6:
Cardio or Rest

Day 7:
Cardio or Rest

Or like this:

Day 1:
Chest

Day 2:
Back

Day 3:
Shoulders

Day 4:
Arms

Day 5:
Chest Weak Point Training & Cardio or Rest

Day 6:
Legs

Day 7:
Cardio or Rest

Either of these schedules would work because your chest is given enough time to recover from the first workout before you perform the second one.

Let's say that you need to address your legs, though, and you currently train them on Fridays. You couldn't do another workout the next day or even on Sunday—this would lead to overtraining. Instead, you'd want to add your weak point training to the beginning or end of your Monday or Tuesday workout, which gives your legs enough time to recover before they are trained again.

Generally speaking, I recommend addressing no more than two weak points at a time or again this can lead to overtraining. (Some people feel everything in their physique is weak and try to train their entire body twice per week with intense workouts and inevitably wind up overtrained.)

If you feel you have more than two weak points that you need to address, then you alternate them, training two on the first week's Weak Point Workout and the other two on the next week's.

You choose exercises according to the principles laid out for the main program. You can do different exercises in your weak point training than those done on your normal days, or not.

For example, my current weak points are my shoulders and lats. My normal workouts are exactly what you see in in the bonus report (I'm currently doing one of those mesocycles), and my weak point training is on day 6, and it currently looks like this:

Myofibrillar Sets
2 x Dumbbell Press
2 x Wide-Grip Lat Pulldown

Sarcoplasmic Sets
2 x Side Lateral Raise
2 x Pull-Ups (weighted)

I've been doing this for several months now and have seen great improvements in both areas. It's simple, and it works.

Don't get overzealous with this workout and try to include Power Sets or more Myofibrillar Sets. This workout should be less intense to avoid overtraining the muscles. Be patient, and the results will come.

10

HOW TO MAINTAIN MUSCLE AND STRENGTH WITH MINIMAL EXERCISE

WE KNOW HOW MUCH PERSISTENCE AND consistency it takes to get a great physique.

You have to hit the weights 3 to 5 times per week, every week, for at least 1 or 2 years. You often have to also find time for a couple of hours of cardio per week. You have to watch what you eat, regulating intake to meet your goals of gaining or losing weight.

While some of us learn to enjoy the process, nobody ever said it was easy. It takes intense, regular work, and above all, consistency.

Now, how do things change once you've achieved the body you desire? Do you have to work just as hard to keep a good physique as you do to build one?

If that question doesn't matter so much to you—if you're like me and you just enjoy the fitness lifestyle—then maybe this one will catch your interest:

How can you maintain muscle and strength when you're not able to follow your regular exercise routine?

Although some of us would love to be able to hit the gym 5 times per week without any unplanned breaks, year-in, year-out…life will inevitably throw us curve balls.

For example, staying in shape while traveling can be tricky. The holidays are notorious for messing with schedules (and diets). Family and work often take precedence over personal time.

Are you simply doomed to losing muscle and strength in such situations? Or is there an easy way to avert such problems?

Well, as you'll see in this chapter, it's much easier than most people think to maintain muscle and strength and even continue to make gains.

Let's get to it.

HOW MUCH EXERCISE IT TAKES TO MAINTAIN MUSCLE AND STRENGTH

I have good news for you:

It's much easier to maintain a good physique and level of conditioning than it is to get there.

How easy, you ask?

Well, consider a study conducted by researchers at the University of Alberta with competitive rowers.[25] After 10 weeks of weightlifting 3 times per week, 18 varsity female rowers were split into two groups. Both groups then did 6 weeks of maintenance resistance training, with one group training once per week and the other twice per week.

The results? Both groups improved their strength in two exercises they performed each week and maintained strength in the four others in their routine.

Yes, that's right. According to that research, you can maintain your strength by training just once per week. And that's not the only study demonstrating this.

Researchers from the University of Alabama at Birmingham conducted a study wherein subjects lifted weights 3 times per week (9 sets per workout) for 5 months, and then they were assigned to 1 of 3 groups for the next 8 months:

1. No exercise at all

2. One weightlifting workout per week that consisted of 9 total sets

3. One weightlifting workout per week that consisted of 3 total sets[26]

Over the course of the following 8 months, group 1 lost muscle (of course), but both groups 2 and 3 were able to maintain most of the muscle they had gained in the first part of the study and even increase their strength.

So, what we can learn from these studies is this: you can not only maintain muscle and strength by training only 1 or 2 times per week, but you can also make gains.

Sure, you won't be able to make the same kinds of gains as you can training 3 to 5 times per week, but you can do better than most people think.

One study conducted by researchers at the University of Queensland showed that subjects who trained a muscle group twice per week made about 70% of the gains of those training 3 times per week.[27]

A study conducted by researchers at the University of Florida showed that subjects doing isometric training twice per week made about 80% of the gains of those training 3 times per week.[28]

Researchers from Laurentian University found that one group of subjects training twice per week, performing 27 total sets per week, made equal gains to another group training 3 times per week for the same number of sets.[29]

The key takeaway here is that weekly workout volume is at least as important, if not more important than, workout frequency.

So, here's the point that will come as a great relief to many:

Regardless of what's going on in your life, if you can sneak away from the hustle and bustle for a couple of hours per week, you can minimally keep your hard-earned gains.

Now, how do you best go about the training? What workouts will deliver the best results when you're only training 1 or 2 times per week?

THE PERFECT MUSCLE MAINTENANCE PROGRAM

When you can only train once or twice per week, what you do is very important.

If you're in decent shape and simply hopped on some machines and got a pump, you certainly won't make gains and will almost certainly lose muscle over time.

The bottom line is when you reduce workout frequency, you have to increase volume and maintain a high level of intensity.

You also want to focus on exercises that recruit the maximum amount of muscle, which are the big compound lifts like Deadlifts, Squats, Bench Press, and Military Press.

Here's how to get the most out of training twice per week.

TRAINING TWICE PER WEEK

When you can only train twice per week, I recommend you use one day to train your push and pull muscles and another day to focus on your legs, with a little additional push.

The following workouts take about an hour to complete. Rest 2 or 3 minutes in between each set, and take at least one day of rest in between each (2 days of rest between each is ideal, I think).

Day 1: Push/Pull

Deadlift: Warm-Up and 3 sets of 4 to 6 reps
Incline Bench Press: Warm-Up and 3 sets of 4 to 6 reps
Barbell Row: 3 sets of 4 to 6 reps
Military Press: 3 sets of 4 to 6 reps

Day 2: Legs and Additional Push

Bench Press: Warm-Up and 3 sets of 4 to 6 reps
Squat: Warm-Up and 3 sets 4 to 6 reps
Hack Squat (sled, not barbell) or Leg Press: 3 sets of 4 to 6 reps
Romanian Deadlift: 3 sets of 4 to 6 reps

These are brutally simple and effective workouts. With them, you can actually make gains, not simply remain the same.

TRAINING ONCE PER WEEK

If you can only train once per week, don't despair. You can minimally maintain muscle, strength, and conditioning, and possibly even make gains.

The following workout hits every major muscle group in the body and also takes about an hour to complete. Rest 2 or 3 minutes in between each set. It's hard, but very effective.

Squat: Warm-Up and 3 sets 4 to 6 reps
Deadlift: Warm-Up and 3 sets 4 to 6 reps
Bench Press: Warm-Up and 3 sets of 4 to 6 reps
Barbell Row: 3 sets of 4 to 6 reps
Military Press: 3 sets of 4 to 6 reps

Again, nothing fancy here: just heavy, compound lifting, hitting your entire body.

So, if you're short on time or just want to cruise and maintain your physique, I hope this chapter helps!

In the next few chapters, I'm going to share you with some extremely helpful tips for improving leg, hip, and shoulder mobility, as the more flexible these parts of your body are, the better you will be able to perform many of the exercises in the *Beyond Bigger Leaner Stronger* program.

11

HOW TO IMPROVE LOWER-BODY FLEXIBILITY AND MOBILITY

IMPAIRED LOWER-BODY FLEXIBILITY AND mobility (the ability to move freely) can seriously mess with your ability to train your legs and back properly. This is mainly because it holds back major exercises like the Squat and Deadlift, which are incredibly effective for training your entire back, lower body, and core, but only if you do them correctly. Half-reps don't count.

And while it's common for gym-goers to sneer at others who do Squats and Deadlifts incorrectly, what they don't realize is many people simply lack the flexibility to perform these exercises properly. They couldn't perform a proper rep even if they wanted to.

The fact is learning proper form for the Squat and Deadlift is tough regardless of your current condition, and the longer people have been half-repping, the harder it will be for them to correct their form. (Repeatedly training a muscle with a limited range of motion reduces flexibility.)[30]

Well, in this chapter, we're going to talk about how we can use hip and ankle flexibility and mobility exercises to help us improve our lower-body training.

HOW TO IMPROVE HIP FLEXIBILITY AND MOBILITY

Lack of hip flexibility is probably the most common problem that prevents people from performing exercises like the Squat and Deadlift properly. This is a matter of hip flexion.

Hip flexion is simply the technical term for a decrease in the angle between the thigh and pelvis. As your knee rises, hip flexion occurs. Several muscles are involved in this action, and if they lack enough flexibility, you will have serious problems with certain exercises.

Fortunately, you can do simple stretching exercises to improve hip flexibility and mobility and thus eliminate the problem.

Now, regarding the exercises, you must keep a few points in mind:

- Don't stretch before your weightlifting as this can increase the risk of shoulder injury. Stretch after your weightlifting or at another time altogether.

- Don't try to push through tightness. Don't approach flexibility exercises like weightlifting—don't try to blast through sticking points, as this can cause injury.

- Stop at tightness, hold for 5 seconds, and release. You have to be patient when you're working on increasing mobility.

- Take it slow at first, especially if you're nursing an injury. Again, building up flexibility takes time and patience, especially if you're recovering from an injury. Even minor strains can take several weeks to fully heal when cared for properly and much longer if continually aggravated.

Alright, let's now take a look at the exercises themselves.

KNEELING HIP FLEXOR STRETCH

This is one of the best stretches for improving hip flexibility.

It allows you to work the bottom position of the Squat one leg at a time, and that's how you want to look at it: squatting one leg a time, and working out tight spots in the bottom position.

The key to getting the most out of this stretch is finding tight spots and then moving in and out of them as opposed to just sitting in them. Work tight spots by oscillating in small circles and rotating and sliding in and out of them, and do this until they release.

You want to keep the foot of your front leg firmly planted on the ground. Remember that you're practicing a proper Squat here, and in a proper Squat, your feet are perfectly flat on the floor.

Here's how to do the stretch:

Your starting position is on your hands and knees, with your right foot next to your right hand, and your right shin at a 90-degree angle to the ground.

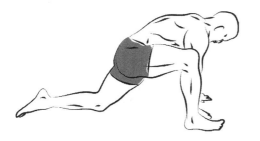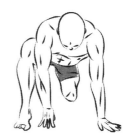

Root your right foot to the ground with your right hand and stretch your left leg back, pushing your hip toward the ground. Flatten your back. Once you're in this position, you can move around, pushing your weight into the corner of your butt until you reach the end of your flexibility range.

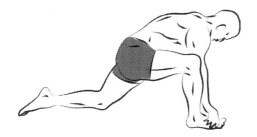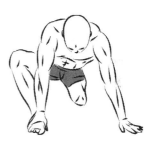

Look for points of tightness by rotating your upper body away from your front leg.

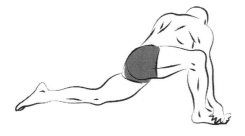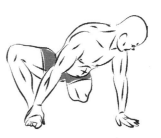

To help with keeping your knees out in your Squats, lower your left elbow to the ground, stick your right foot to the ground with your left hand, turn your upper body toward your front leg, and push your knee out using your right hand.

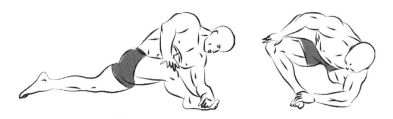

Work on this for 2 to 3 minutes per leg, and then move on to the next stretch below.

PSOAS QUAD STRETCH

The psoas major is a pelvic muscle that plays a key role in hip flexion. When this muscle is too tight, squatting properly is basically impossible.

I ran into this problem years ago when I finally fixed my Squat form, and I had to do a lot of psoas stretching in addition to regular squatting to finally handle it.

One of the stretches that helped is a simple psoas quad stretch. Here's how to do it:

Start with your feet against a vertical, flat surface like a box, couch, or wall.

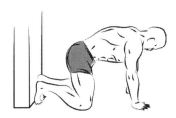

Move your left leg back and fit your knee into the corner. Position your shin so it's flush with the surface.

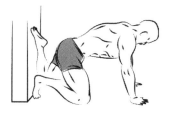

Squeeze your left glute and move your right foot into a vertical position. If you can't reach this position, bring your right leg as far as you can and move in and out of the range. You can also position a small box, coffee table, or chair in front of you to lean on for extra stability.

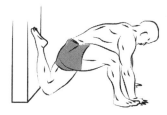

With your butt still squeezed, push your hips toward the ground. This is probably going to be uncomfortable, so take it easy. Remain in this position for a minute or two.

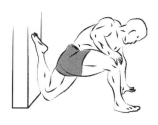

Perform this drive and release pattern for 2 to 3 minutes for each leg.

YOUR WEEKLY HIP FLEXIBILITY AND MOBILITY ROUTINE

Do these two stretches 3 or 4 times per week and you should notice a dramatic improvement within 4 to 6 weeks.

HOW TO IMPROVE
ANKLE FLEXIBILITY AND MOBILITY

Ankle tightness can prevent you from being able to properly drop into the bottom of a Squat, with the weight solidly on your heels, your chest up, and spine in a neutral position.

If your heels want to lift off the ground when you're squatting or if you tend to shift the weight forward onto your toes and have trouble dropping your butt down to the parallel position or lower, then ankle tightness is likely the problem.

To improve your ankle flexibility and mobility, you can mash up and stretch the tissues of your feet, ankles, and calves. Here are two good ways to do this.

PLANTAR BALL SMASH

The plantar fascia is a sheet of connective tissue on the bottom of your foot, and when it becomes aggravated or stiff, it can cause ankle and lower leg tightness, and in more severe cases, become really painful.

Fortunately, it's easy to resolve. This solution requires a hard ball that still has some give so you can avoid tissue damage (I like to use a lacrosse ball).

All you want to do is stand on the ball barefoot and roll your foot over it from ball to heel, looking for hot spots. Once you hit a tender spot, hold pressure on it, applying pressure and releasing. You can even do this while sitting (but to really get pressure, you'll have to stand).

FOAM ROLLER CALF SMASH

With the average athletic person taking more than 5,000 steps per day, the calves take quite a beating.

If you walk with your feet turned out or wear the wrong types of shoes, the calves can get really tight, and that tightness can ripple down into the heel. This, in turn, kills ankle mobility and can lead to serious problems like bone spurs and Achilles tendonitis.

An easy way to start working out calf tightness is to use a foam roller on it. We're going to talk more about foam rolling in a couple of chapters, but I want to include this exercise here. This is a light approach, but it can definitely give some relief.

Here's how it works:

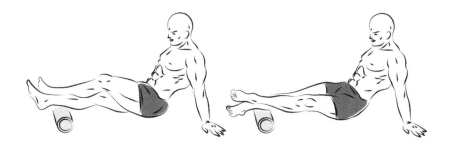

As you can see, the position is very simple: you place one calf and Achilles tendon on the roller and cross your other leg over it to add pressure. You then roll your under leg side to side, finding spots to press into and release as you move up the calf.

If you have a friend to help, you can really dig in, getting a lot more pressure into your calf than you can apply alone.

Again, the procedure is the same: have your friend apply as much pressure as you can take, and roll your leg side to side, moving up the calf, finding and clearing tight spots.

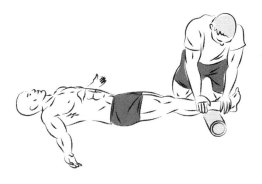

YOUR WEEKLY ANKLE FLEXIBILITY AND MOBILITY ROUTINE

Do these exercises 3 to 4 times per week, either before or after your hip work.

HOW TO DRILL IN PROPER SQUAT FORM

As you improve your hip and ankle flexibility and mobility, you'll find it easier and easier to do Squats properly.

To get the Squat form down so perfectly that you don't even have to think about it, I recommend you do the following Squat drill at the end of each of your flexibility and mobility sessions.

It will not only teach you proper form through repetition, but it will also show you how much the stretching exercises are helping.

WALL SQUAT

The Wall Squat is a great Squat form drill. It's very simple but can be quite a challenge to do properly:

- Face the wall with your toes a few inches from it and feet shoulder-width apart and turned slightly out.

- Fully extend your arms above your head and place your palms against the wall, arms parallel to each other.

- Push your hips back and lower yourself down into a full Squat position (or as low as you can go), with your hands remaining on the wall. Don't allow your head, knees, or torso to touch the wall.

- Focus on keeping your knees in line with your toes (pushed out) and your chest up. Keep your spine in a neutral position (don't overarch or round it).

- If your head, knees, or torso touch the wall, stop at this point, fix your form, and hold the position. Move around a bit to get a good stretch.

If you start doing weekly flexibility and mobility exercises for your squatting, you should see a rapid and dramatic improvement in your workouts.

12

HOW TO IMPROVE SHOULDER FLEXIBILITY AND MOBILITY

INFLEXIBLE SHOULDERS GET IN THE WAY of quite a few of your major lifts: namely the Squat, Military Press, and Bench Press.

Shoulder pain, problems, and injuries are also prevalent among weightlifters, primarily due to improper form on the Bench Press and Shoulder Press variants and an imbalance between chest and back training. (Many guys focus too much on their chest training and neglect their backs, which results in the pectorals pulling the shoulders down and inward, setting you up for injury.)

Fortunately, you can overcome shoulder pain and inflexibility easily if you address it properly.

Regardless of whether you're new to lifting or experienced or whether you're currently experiencing shoulder problems, I recommend that you start doing these stretching exercises every week. If you're currently dealing with shoulder impairments, they will improve symptoms; if you're not, they will help you maintain optimal shoulder health and function as well as prevent future injury.

Before we get to the flexibility and mobility routine, though, let's assess your current level of shoulder flexibility.

A SIMPLE SHOULDER FLEXIBILITY TEST

An easy way to test your shoulder flexibility is to try to get into the following position:

If you get into the arms-up position and someone at your side can't see your eyes and at least some of your ear (if your arm is in the way and you can't move it back enough to reveal your ear), your training will benefit greatly from improving your shoulder flexibility.

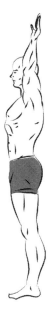

HOW TO IMPROVE SHOULDER FLEXIBILITY

If you're lacking shoulder flexibility, you should focus on two things to improve it:

1. Ensure you're not neglecting your back muscles in your training, as an imbalance between chest and back development is the most common cause of shoulder problems.

2. Do shoulder flexibility exercises several times per week.

If you do both of these things, you can get rid of nagging shoulder issues you might be dealing with and prevent them if you're not currently having any problems.

Many of us spend long periods in the car and sitting at a desk with our shoulders rolled forward. This can result in very tight shoulders that get locked in an unstable position, which can then compromise your training.

Alright, let's get to the exercises.

ANTERIOR DELTOID SMASH

This exercise requires the use of a lacrosse or similar (hard rubber) ball, but it is one of my favorite mobilization techniques for the anterior deltoid.

Here's the area you target with the ball:

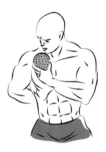

And here's what you do:

With your arm behind your back, position yourself so the ball is in the target area.

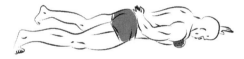

Use your other arm to push yourself off the ground, rotate toward this arm, and work the tissues, applying pressure in waves.

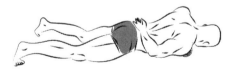

Once you find a sore spot, you can apply more pressure by locking your hands behind your back.

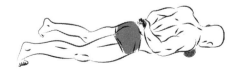

SHOULDER DISLOCATIONS

Don't worry: this exercise doesn't result in dislocated shoulders.

It's a great all-around shoulder mobility exercise and very simple to do. All you need is a long broomstick (or something similar).

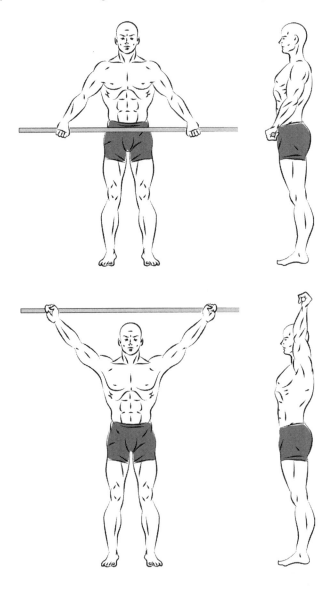

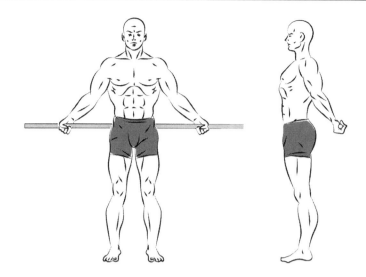

Keep your spine neutral, squeeze your glutes, and stand nice and tall—root yourself to the ground. You don't want your hips moving forward or backward; you want to stand perfectly upright and keep your hips still.

You also want to keep your shoulders back and down. Don't hunch your shoulders on the way up and relax them on the way down.

The tightness of your shoulders will dictate how wide your grip needs to be. The tighter they are, the wider you'll need to make your grip. As your flexibility improves, however, you will be able to gradually narrow your grip.

Flexible people will be able to perform the exercise with their hands at less than two shoulder-widths apart.

DOUBLE-ARM SHOULDER STRETCH

This stretch is great for working out anything that is tight in your shoulders. All you need is a horizontal pole or surface you can grab onto.

Grab onto the bar or surface with your palm facing down.

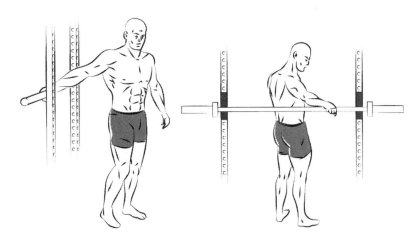

Grab onto the bar with your other arm, placing your hands as close together as possible without compromising the position.

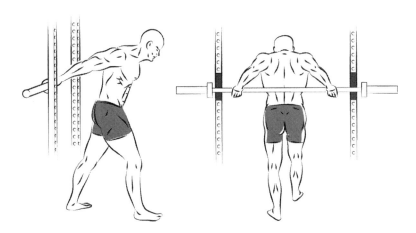

If you can take more pressure, lower your body with the goal of bringing your shoulders to the height of your shoulders without having to break the position.

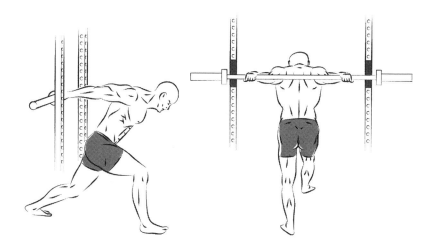

You can also do a one-arm variant of this stretch by grabbing onto a pole or even a doorframe.

YOUR WEEKLY SHOULDER FLEXIBILITY ROUTINE

A good place to start your routine is to perform 2 sets of 10 reps, with 60 seconds of rest in between each set. Do this twice per week. As your flexibility improves, you can add more exercises and/or sets as desired.

Here's what I do twice per week:

• 5 minutes of Anterior Deltoid Smash (about 2.5 minutes per side)

• 2 sets of 20 Shoulder Dislocations

• 5 minutes of Double-Arm Shoulder Stretch

This keeps my shoulders flexible and the joint tight and in alignment. I rarely experience shoulder pain or problems and have been strain-free for years now (knock on wood).

13

HOW TO USE THE FOAM ROLLER TO IMPROVE PERFORMANCE

FOAM ROLLING USED TO BE A mysterious, "experimental" technique used solely by professional athletes, coaches, and therapists, with its ultimate effectiveness unproven.

Well, thanks to years of technique development and recent clinical research, foam rolling has become a common practice for people at all levels of fitness, and for good reason.

For no more than $40 and 5 to 10 minutes of your time a few days per week, you can use foam rolling to dramatically improve mobility and thus range of motion, to reduce the risk of injury, and to remove pain that you might experience while you put your body through certain motions.

I introduced you to foam rolling in the chapter on improving lower-body mobility, and in this chapter, I want to explain why foam rolling works and show you five of my favorite foam rolling exercises for supporting my weightlifting routine.

HOW FOAM ROLLING WORKS

In fancy-speak, foam rolling is a self-myofascial release method that relaxes overactive muscles that prevent proper activation and motion.

To understand self-myofascial release, let's break it down:

Myo- is a prefix meaning muscle, and fascia is a soft, fibrous tissue that surrounds muscles, blood vessels, and nerves, allowing for mobility while providing support and protection.

Thus, self-myofascial release simply refers to a way you can release tension in the fascia surrounding your muscles and the muscles themselves.

You see, fascia can become overly tight through overuse, injury, and even inactivity. The result is inflammation, pain, muscle tension, reduction of blood flow, and loss of mobility, and if the problem becomes severe or prolonged, the fascia can thicken, causing pain and further inflammation.[31]

Now, mechanically speaking, foam rolling is very simple.

You position your body in certain ways on a foam cylindrical tube to put pressure on trigger points, which are tight spots in muscles that, when pressed on, produce pain that refers to other areas in the body (you can feel pain in areas other than where you're applying pressure) .

By holding pressure on these trigger points, your body will gradually relax the areas, causing the pain to fade.[32] This is known as releasing trigger points.

"Relaxation" is underselling the benefits of foam rolling, though. It can make quite a difference in your training.

THE BENEFITS OF FOAM ROLLER EXERCISES

When you release fascial and muscular tightness, inflammation and pain diminish, and blood flow is restored.[33] [34]

While this might sound nice, it means a lot for us athletes.

For example, a study conducted by researchers from the Memorial University of Newfoundland found that foam rolling increases range of motion without decreasing strength (which is a problem with pre-workout stretching).[35]

The greater the range of motion in an exercise, the more work your muscles have to do, which in turn leads to greater gains in strength and size.[36] And because it doesn't impair performance, you can foam roll before a workout to prime your body for the training.[37]

A study conducted by researchers at Osaka Aoyama University found that foam rolling reduces arterial stiffness and thus improves blood flow.[38]

Better blood flow means better removal of metabolic waste (toxic substances left over from various cellular functions) from tissues and better delivery of nutrients, which ultimately helps with muscle repair.

We can see these effects in a study that demonstrated that foam rolling reduces the severity of delayed-onset muscle soreness (DOMS) that occurs after training and increases your range of motion.[39]

So, as you can see, regular foam rolling over longer periods of time can make quite a difference in the results you get out of your training.

HOW TO FOAM ROLL PROPERLY

The wrong way to foam roll is to just roll a large muscle group up and down, applying light to moderate pressure.

The right way to foam roll is to move slowly over the tissues, back and forth, applying deep pressure. When you find painful spots, you stick on them, moving in and out, applying heavy pressure in waves. You continue until the pain subsides and then move on to find another spot.

When done properly, foam rolling can be very uncomfortable, but it also produces great results.

MY THREE FAVORITE FOAM ROLLER EXERCISES

You can do a wide variety of foam roller exercises, but here are my top three.

You can perform these exercises pre-workout to improve performance, post-workout to improve recovery, or both, or at any other time you want.

In terms of time, I like to spend a couple of minutes on each, finding and releasing one or two trigger points for each muscle group.

QUAD AND ILIOTIBIAL TRACT (IT BAND) FOAM ROLLER EXERCISE

The IT band runs along the outer side of your leg, and its associated muscles are involved in various hip movements and in stabilizing the knees.

Regular, proper squatting will often create trigger points in the IT band, which in turn impair range of motion and performance.

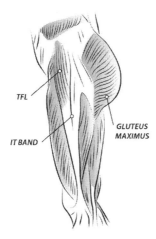

The quads are a major muscle group in the leg, and they can get tight from regular training and then shorter from too much sitting.

With this foam roller exercise, you can work out the tension of both.

Lie over the foam roller on your side, using the leg not being rolled and your upper body to support your weight.

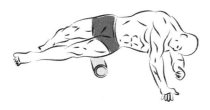

Slowly rotate around in the direction of facing the ground.

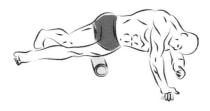

Once you're facing the ground, place the leg not being rolled next to the one you're working on and move up and down, finding tight spots.

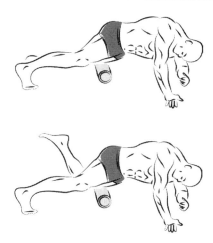

Bring the heel of the leg being worked off the ground toward your butt. Continue to rotate and move the area up and down.

Once there are no more pain spots, move a few inches up the muscle and repeat, finding and clearing out tight spots.

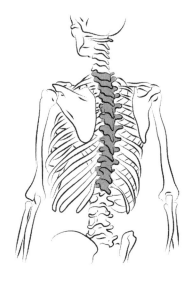

THORACIC SPINE FOAM ROLLER EXERCISE

The thoracic spine is the middle segment of the spine; in humans, it consists of 12 vertebrae.

This region of the body has major back muscles that can get very tight with training and can get aggravated by sitting at a desk all day (the rhomboids in particular).

This foam roller exercise helps you release tension in the area and loosen up the tissues.

The key to this exercise, like other foam roller exercises, is producing a smashing force by arching and relaxing your back. Don't just lightly roll back and forth.

Wrap your arms around your body and position yourself so the roller is at the bottom of your ribcage (the last vertebrae of the thoracic spine). By bear hugging yourself, you "unwrap" the muscles of your back so they can be targeted.

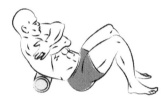

Arch your back, holding your bear hug tight. Extend as far as you can, applying more and more pressure to the area.

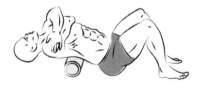

Maintaining the bear hug and your weight on the roller, sit up, shift your butt a little toward your feet, and arch and extend.

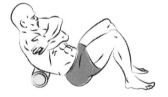 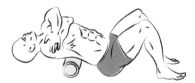

Repeat this process until you've worked all the way up your spine to the base of your neck.

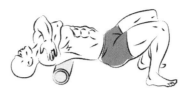

When you find tight spots, you can help work them out by rolling from side to side.

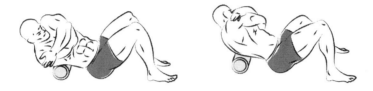

If you notice that one side is particularly tight, you can remain on that side and roll the tight area up and down.

LATISSIMUS DORSI FOAM ROLLER EXERCISE

The latissimus dorsi, or lat, is another muscle primarily targeted in back training, and thus it often develops trigger points.

The foam roller exercise for it is very simple.

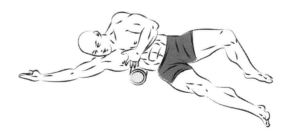

Lie on your side with one leg extended and one planted and with the roller at the bottom of your lat. Slide down the roller, working out tight spots as you encounter them.

BUYING A FOAM ROLLER

A good foam roller is moderately dense. If the foam is too soft, you can't apply enough pressure; if it's too hard, you can wind up bruising yourself, causing too much trauma to the trigger point areas.

There are a few foam rollers in particular that I like, and you'll find links to buy them in the bonus report at the end of this book.

I recommend that you foam roll regularly while on the program. It will help tremendously with maintaining proper form and warding off nagging aches and pains.

WANT MORE MOBILITY?

If you like the mobility work I've laid out in the last couple of chapters and want more, then I highly recommend you read Dr. Kelly Starrett's *Becoming a Supple Leopard.*

It's the Bible of mobility and contains a wealth of powerful, practical advice. It will show you how to fix poor lifting mechanics that reduce power, how to improve athletic performance, how to prevent and rehabilitate common injuries, how to restore function to joints, and much more.

14

HOW TO BREAK THROUGH WEIGHTLIFTING PLATEAUS

NOTHING IS MORE FRUSTRATING THAN HITTING a seemingly unbreakable weightlifting plateau.

You know the rub: every day, you hit the gym hopped up on pre-workout drink and attitude, determined to push more weight than your last workout. You load the plates, turn your music up loud, convince yourself it's light weight, and hit the set with everything you've got... and it quickly humbles you. It feels damn heavy, and you end up doing exactly what you've been doing every week (or worse).

What gives? And what can you do to finally make progress again? Let's find out.

THE PHYSIOLOGY OF PROGRESS

The human body is incredibly good at adapting to stimuli, and regardless of whether we're talking metabolism or muscle mass, its goal is to maintain a normalized state wherein things more or less stay the same (homeostasis).

This is great for survival but not so great for building muscle and strength. As time goes on, the body gets better and better at adapting to training, and this is why many people fall into a rut: they simply don't exert enough effort to progress. The bottom line is once your newbie gains are behind you, you have to work damn hard to force your muscles to continue growing larger and stronger.

Physiologically speaking, what you're going for is known as *supercompensation*. This is the process whereby the body augments existing muscle fibers, tendons, and ligaments to become bigger and stronger.

As you know, the primary factor driving supercompensation is progressive overload—lifting more weight for a given rep range over time. This is why a plateau in size is always accompanied by a plateau in strength. Rest assured that people who look the same month after month are lifting more or less the same weights month after month as well.

And this is why you want to avoid plateaus at all costs. If each week's workouts are exact duplicates of each other—if you're doing the same exercises with the same weights and for the same number of reps—you will be able to maintain your current physique and performance levels, but you won't progress toward better a better state.

Now, a properly designed program and dietary regimen go far toward preventing plateaus. I don't run into too many people who plateau on my programs. Nevertheless, plateaus are part of the game. They happen to everyone, even if infrequently, and even on the best of programs. So don't despair when it happens to you. Patiently use the strategies in this chapter to break through these sticking points, and you'll never fall into a real rut.

So, let's get started, first by defining what a plateau is.

WHAT A PLATEAU IS AND ISN'T

Whenever people tell me they're stuck on a program, I always ask for the details first. What do they mean, exactly?

Often, it turns out they are making progress; they just aren't making the type of progress they want to see (they aren't adding weight as quickly as they once were, or they aren't improving on all exercises they perform in each workout).

I then explain what I want to explain to you here, which has to do with expectations and benchmarks.

Unless you're new to weightlifting, you will not be able to add weight to the bar every week and maintain proper form and rep ranges. Instead, your weekly goal for each workout should be to increase at least one of your lifts by 1 or 2 reps, and it will usually be your first exercise.

For example, if you deadlifted 455 pounds last week for 2 reps, your goal is to get 3 to 4 reps this week (and you probably won't get 4). If you do that and the rest of your workout is exactly the same as last week's (same weight and reps for each subsequent exercise), that's a successful workout. I know that might sound odd, but just increasing 1 or 2 reps on one exercise is enough to induce supercompensation, and you should be happy.

Based on my experience in my own training and working with hundreds of people, if your body is ready to progress, you'll probably see an improvement in more than just one exercise of your workout, but sometimes it's just that first big compound lift that improves, and the rest stays the same. Other times it's the first set or two of the second exercise. Less often, the improvement could come in one of your Sarcoplasmic Sets. Regardless of how you improve, any progress means you're not stuck in a plateau.

A true plateau is the situation where every lift in a workout is stuck at a certain weight for a certain number of reps for at least 3 weeks. That is, lifting the same amount of weight for each exercise for the same number of reps for at least 3 weeks in a row. If that happens, it's time to address it with one or more of the strategies below.

COULD IT BE TECHNIQUE OR MOBILITY?

Improper form can kill progress, especially on the big, important lifts like the Squat, Deadlift, and Bench Press. If your setup or execution is off, you will plateau at some point, and if you try to power through it, you may get hurt.

If I'm stuck (and from time to time even when things are going well), I like to have someone video me while I'm performing each exercise so I can review my form. I'll put the videos on my computer and blow them up big so I can see what's going on. And more than once I've discovered something obviously wrong in my form that, when corrected, enabled me to progress again.

For example, several months ago, I found I tended to lean too far forward in my squats when the weight got heavy, which was putting too much stress on my hip flexors. This was preventing me from moving up in weight. To correct this, I backed down on the weight to give my hip flexors a break and work on my form. Within a month or so, I was rapidly moving up again, this time with proper form and no hip flexor pains.

Sometimes correcting technique is trickier, though. And it almost always is due to mobility problems.

As you know, impaired upper- and lower-body mobility can seriously compromise form. Some people simply can't perform certain exercises correctly because their body can't do the movements. Fortunately, this too is fairly simple to correct. The mobility routines I've given in this book, if done regularly, are enough to handle most problems.

MAKE SURE YOU'RE GETTING ENOUGH SLEEP

If you don't sleep enough, your body just won't be able to perform at its best. And when you're demanding a lot from it in the gym, getting adequate rest every night is especially important for both recovery and performance.

People have known this anecdotally for some time, but research backs it up. One study restricted the sleep of eight males aged 18 to 24 to three hours per night for three successive nights and found that their strength on the Bench Press, Leg Press, and Deadlift was significantly compromised and the workouts were much more fatiguing than usual.[40]

While that's a rather extreme example of sleep deprivation, other research has shown that milder amounts of sleep restriction also compromise performance and the body's ability to recover from exercise.[41] Research has also shown that extending sleep to a minimum of 10 hours in bed each night increases physical performance (subjects felt better mentally, ran faster, shot basketballs more accurately, and were able to exercise longer before feeling fatigued).[42]

Now, that doesn't mean we should all sleep 10 hours or more each night. In fact, studies have shown that only a small percentage of people actually need that much sleep.[43] But we should give our body as much sleep as it needs, and according to the National Sleep Foundation, adults need 7 to 9 hours of sleep per night to avoid the negative effects of sleep deprivation. A small percentage of people do fine with less, and a small percentage need more.

Since genetics and age affect how much sleep your body needs, a simple way to determine what's optimal for you is to pick a two-week period such as a vacation and go to bed at the same time each night without an alarm set.

Chances are, you'll sleep longer than usual at first if you have "sleep debt" to cancel out, but toward the end of the second week, your body will establish a pattern of sleeping about the same amount every night. And it's trying to tell you something: that's exactly how much sleep it needs. Stick to that, and you'll never battle with the effects of sleep deprivation.

ARE YOU BECOMING OVERTRAINED?

Overtraining can be insidious, especially in its beginning phases, when its symptoms are mild and hard to recognize.

When overtraining begins to set in, the first things to falter will be your strength and muscle endurance. Your workouts just start feeling hard, no matter what you do. This is nothing more than an accumulation of central nervous system fatigue, and it's easy to handle (a Rest or Deload Week).

If you're a week or two away from your planned Rest or Deload Week and you're stuck and everything feels unusually heavy, it's very likely that you just need to rest or deload a little early, and you'll come back ready to progress again.

However, if you come back from your rest or deloading and remain stuck, you know it's not an overtraining issue. If you're only a couple of weeks into a mesocycle and you're stuck, it's likely not an overtraining issue.

GIVE YOUR WORKOUTS
EVERYTHING YOU'VE GOT

Following a program like *Beyond Bigger Leaner Stronger* doesn't just require physical toughness; it requires mental toughness as well. Squatting, deadlifting, and pressing hundreds of pounds over and over isn't for the lazy or weak willed.

Sometimes people fall into a rut simply because they don't hit their workouts with everything they've got. Their minds are elsewhere, and they're just going through the motions. We've all experienced this before, and it doesn't take much to snap out of it once we recognize the problem.

Sometimes external factors are working against us. You know, the overly chatty or lazy workout partner, the tranquilizing gym music, the time of day (some people are noticeably stronger and more energetic later in the afternoon than early in the morning), or the nursing of an injury, even if mild.

The solutions to such problems are simple, of course. Let the Chatty Cathy know that while you have nothing against socializing, too much of it detracts from your workouts. Get an iPod and fire up music that gets your heart racing. Work out when you feel strongest and most energetic. Be patient with injuries and make sure they're fully healed before you go full bore again.

There are often inner obstacles to overcome as well. Sometimes we psych ourselves out when trying to hit heavier weights, sometimes we're too critical of ourselves, and sometimes we're just in a bad mood or don't want to be in the gym.

These problems can be easily brushed aside as well. Psyching yourself up for a lift or workout is just as easy as psyching yourself out: you can create your emotions at will. Get fired up. Get ready to give it everything you've got. Visualize yourself hitting the lift perfectly. You don't have to stomp around the gym like a raging bull, but don't worry if you look a little "too into it." You're there to get results, not to impress others with your cool, calm demeanor.

When you're in the gym, allow yourself the luxury of temporarily letting go of whatever other problems you're dealing with in life. Nothing is going to fall apart in the hour you spend moving heavy stuff. Keep your mind on the muscles being trained, the next rep, and the next set. Think of it as your meditation time.

USING DIET TO BREAK THROUGH PLATEAUS

In many cases, a plateau in weight, size, and strength is caused by nothing more than not eating enough. And for some people, "enough" is quite a lot.

For example, I regularly e-mail with guys weighing 170 to 180 pounds who need to eat upward of 4,000 to even 5,000 calories per day just to gain about 1 pound per week. In most cases, these guys are new to weightlifting, which makes that even more unusual.

As you get bigger and stronger, the amount of food that you'll need to eat to continue getting bigger and stronger will likely go up. Just as you slowly reduce calorie intake when cutting, you often need to slowly increase calorie intake while trying to maximize muscle growth.

So increasing calorie intake is an easy way to get your numbers, both weight and strength, moving up. All you have to do is increase your daily intake by about 100 calories (I prefer increasing my pre- or post-workout carbs by about 25 grams) and reassess after a couple of weeks. If that unsticks you, then keep your calories there for the next few weeks and see how your body responds. If you're progressing again, great; continue until you're not, and then increase intake again.

I've known quite a few people who would start to bulk around 3,000 calories per day and end at over 4,000 calories per day due to gradual increases necessary to continue making progress. This is a good thing. It means your metabolism is healthy, and when you start cutting to strip away the fat you've gained, you'll be able to eat quite a bit of food as you can gradually work your calories downward from that pinnacle.

CUT BACK ON THE CARDIO

Cardio can both hurt and help muscle growth.

It helps by improving insulin sensitivity (which refers to how responsive your cells are to insulin's signals) which in turn improves your body's ability to use nutrients to build muscle, and by improving muscle recovery via increased blood flow.[44][45]

However, it can get in the way of muscle growth in several ways. First, it burns calories that you will need to replace if you are to maintain a small energy surplus, and second, it places additional stress on the body, which can contribute to overtraining.

This is why research has shown that the more cardio you do and the more intense that cardio is, the more your strength and growth will be negatively affected.[46] This is especially true for the "hardgainer" types who have trouble gaining size.

This is why I recommend that you do no more than 2 to 3 cardio sessions per week when you're focusing on building muscle and that you keep each session shorter than 30 minutes. And if you hit a plateau, don't be afraid to drop cardio altogether for a few weeks while you unstick yourself. You can then add it back in once you're moving again.

STRETCH THE REP RANGE OR INCREASE THE WEIGHT IN SMALLER INCREMENTS

Sometimes you'll hit the top of a given rep range, increase the weight a standard amount (10 pounds, whether by moving up 5 pounds in dumbbells or adding 5 pounds to each side of the bar), and fail to hit the bottom of the range on the next set.

For instance, you might Military Press 185 pounds for 6 reps, then move up to 195 pounds for your next set and only get 2 to 3 reps.

You have two options when this happens: you can work with the original weight until you can do a couple of additional reps over the top of the rep range (which should give you what you need to successfully move up), or you can increase the weight in smaller increments using smaller plates. Both work well, and it's a matter of personal preference. I would rather add a little bit of weight than reps, but that's me.

For example, you can drop back to 185 pounds and work with that until you can get 8 reps, or you can use smaller plates to move up to 190 pounds, or even less.

In terms of the *Beyond Bigger Leaner Stronger* program, I like to use this strategy on the Power and Myofibrillar Sets but not the Sarcoplasmic Sets. You have more energy for the Power and Myofibrillar Sets, and the higher rep range of the Sarcoplasmic Sets just isn't as helpful for breaking through a plateau.

If you also prefer adding smaller amounts of weight ("microloading," as it's called), then you'll like the products produced by a company called PlateMates. It offers small, magnetic plates ranging from 5/8 of a pound to 5 pounds, and you can attach them to dumbbells, Olympic bars, larger plates, and even stack-weight machines.

INCREASE THE WEIGHT
AND SEE WHETHER IT STICKS

If you're stuck one rep short of the top of a rep range and you're struggling to hit it so you can move up, sometimes it's worth just giving it a shot. You'll get a rep or two less than you should on your next set, but you can give your body another week or two with that new, heavier weight to see whether it will adapt.

For example, let's say you're working in the 4 to 6 rep range on Squats and you're stuck at 375 pounds for 5 reps. You can move up to 380 pounds, which will probably drop you to 3 reps for your next set (one short of where you'd like to be). The next week, however, you load up 380 again and see whether you can now get 4 reps, and the next week 5 reps, and so forth.

If, after trying this new weight for 2 to 3 weeks, you're still stuck a rep or two short of the bottom of your rep range, then you should move back to the previous weight and use the other strategies in this chapter.

Again, I like to use this strategy on my Power and Myofibrillar Sets but not my Sarcoplasmic Sets.

INCORPORATE REST-PAUSE TRAINING

As you know, I'm not a fan of fancy set schemes like supersets, drop sets, and giant sets, nor am I a fan of nontraditional training protocols like super-slow training, super-fast training, negatives, and the like. Many have been scientifically proven to be no more effective than traditional set schemes and rep rhythms, and my experience is in line with the research (I used to do all kinds of fancy stuff and made poor progress with it).

That said, there is one "special" type of training that has both anecdotal and scientific evidence on its side, and that's the Rest-Pause Set. This is an old school powerlifting method for breaking through plateaus, and researchers from the University of Western Sydney recently studied it. They found it to be an effective way to increase strength via greater muscle fiber recruitment.[47]

The Rest-Pause Set is very simple. You perform an exercise to failure (the point where you can't get another rep without help) and then rest for a short period before performing the exercise to failure again, followed by a short rest, and another set to failure, and so forth.

If you've hit a plateau or just want to try this method of training, turn each of your sets into Rest-Pause Sets for one or two workouts, and then go back to your normal training and see whether that has unstuck you. Here's how to turn the normal sets of *Beyond Bigger Leaner Stronger* into Rest-Pause Sets:

REST-PAUSE TRAINING FOR POWER SETS

Use your normal weight for Power Sets and rest 45 to 60 seconds in between your sets. You'll probably get 2 reps on your first set, 1 on your second set, and 1 rep in each subsequent set (if you're doing more Power Sets, such as in the case of the Power Week).

REST-PAUSE TRAINING FOR MYOFIBRILLAR SETS

Again, use your normal weight and rest 20 to 30 seconds in between your sets. Remember to go to failure each set, even if your reps drop to 2 or 1.

REST-PAUSE TRAINING FOR SARCOPLASMIC SETS

Use your normal weight and rest 10 to 20 seconds in between your sets, going to failure each time.

That's it. Rest-Pause workouts are hard, but they can shatter plateaus.

CHOOSING STRATEGIES TO USE TO BREAK THROUGH PLATEAUS

When I hit a plateau, I move through the above strategies in the order given.

- First, I make sure that my technique and mobility aren't holding me back, that I'm getting enough sleep, and that I'm not overtrained.

- If those things aren't the problem, I make sure that my mind is in the game and that I'm giving my workouts everything I've got.

- If that doesn't resolve it, I assess my diet and may or may not increase my calorie intake (by now I have a very good feel for my body and when more food will or won't do it).

- If diet isn't the issue, I'll cut back on my cardio for a couple of weeks and see whether that unsticks me.

- If it doesn't, I'll try stretching the rep ranges and/or increasing the weight in smaller increments.

- If I'm still stuck after a few weeks of that, I'll do a couple of weeks of Rest-Pause training. I put this last on the list because, in most cases, it's unnecessary. I view it as a last resort, and you'll almost always fix it before getting there.

Once you've hit and broken through a few plateaus, you'll get a good feel for what works best for your body. For me, it's usually related to not sleeping or eating enough or to overtraining. And if it's none of those things, stretching rep ranges and increasing by smaller increments fixes it. Other bodies are different, however, and you'll learn the best way to overcome plateaus through experience.

15

AN INTRODUCTION TO ADVANCED NUTRITION STRATEGIES

NOW THAT WE'VE FULLY COVERED THE training portion of the *Beyond Bigger Leaner Stronger* program, let's dive into dieting.

I'm going to assume you already know the basics covered in *BLS*, such as…

- Maintaining a high-protein diet is essential.

- Eating plenty of nutritious foods is important.

- Keeping your intake of carbohydrates moderately high and your intake of fat moderately low is best for maximizing performance in the gym.

- When we're talking about body composition (building muscle and/or losing fat), how much you eat is much more important than what you eat. Calorie deficits are used to lose fat ("cutting"), and calorie surpluses are used to maximize muscle growth ("bulking").

- With the exception of pre- and post-workout nutrition, meal timing doesn't help you lose fat or build muscle more effectively. Work your meal frequency around your preferences and lifestyle.

- The number of meals you eat per day also doesn't matter. Do what you like most.

In short, I'm going to assume that you know how to gain or lose weight or maintain your weight and that you know how to prepare and follow proper meal plans.

In this section of the book, we're going to look at the nutrition side of the game in a different, more specialized light—one that is more likely to relate to your current or near-future circumstances as an advanced weightlifter.

We're not going to talk about bulking in this book, because there's not much more to say about it beyond what's laid out in *BLS*. Keep your body in a mild calorie surplus, and you'll maximize muscle growth while also gaining some body fat.

While the newbie has to spend the majority of his first couple of years bulking if he wants to build that important foundation of size and strength, the advanced lifter can be more flexible. He can bulk if he wants to get bigger or just enjoy food for a bit, or he can maintain a lean physique for extended periods while still making slow gains in muscle and strength.

This last bit—getting lean and maintaining it—is going to be the focus of the nutrition section of this book.

Specifically, our discussion of nutrition is going to focus on three goals:

1. How to get extremely lean (5 to 7% body fat) without sacrificing a bunch of muscle

2. How to maintain a very lean physique for extended periods without becoming a starved, deprived hermit (yes, you can have a social life and eat tasty food)

3. How to focus on building muscle while still staying lean (under 10% body fat)

These three points are what set apart mediocre physiques from great ones.

The guys with impressive physiques not only have the hard, dense muscle that comes with years of proper training, but they know how to get shredded to show it off and how to stay that way for months at a time.

After we cover those three points in detail, we're going to talk about some different dietary protocols that you've probably heard and wondered about: namely, flexible dieting (or "If It Fits Your Macros" as some call it), intermittent fasting, carb cycling, and Paleo.

But before we start, I want to reiterate a point I've made in previous books and in many articles I've written. You probably already know it well, but it's worth repeating.

The absolute unalterable foundation of proper diet boils down to energy in vs. energy out and to eating proper ratios of protein, carbs, and fat.

It doesn't matter what dietary protocol you use or how fancy you try to get—you simply can't change that fact.

You can't effectively (and naturally) build muscle when you're in a calorie deficit unless you're new to weightlifting (more on exactly why soon), you can't lose fat when you're in a calorie surplus, and you can't "hack" your metabolism by eating exotic nuts or drinking coffee laden with gobs of fat.

What you can do, however, is use the information you're going to learn in this section of the book to optimize your nutrition to make it as effective and comfortable as possible. This section will build on the non-negotiable fundamentals of proper dieting that you learned in *BLS* and the simple dietary regimen that accompanies them.

Think of this section as a toolbox. Each chapter will give you a new tool that can help you fine-tune your nutrition to best meet your needs. Some of the tools will be useful to you, and others probably won't. And that's totally fine.

So, let's get started with the first step of getting shredded without sacrificing your health or sanity: ensuring your metabolism is ready for it.

16

THE SCIENCE OF METABOLIC SPEED AND LOSING OR GAINING WEIGHT

HAVE YOU EVER WONDERED HOW SOME people can eat very little food, exercise a ton, and not lose fat? What is going on exactly? And what should they do? Should they suck it up and eat even less? Push through another hour or two of grueling exercise each week? Or do they need to do something else?

Well, in this chapter, I'm going to break it all down and show you why preserving your metabolic health is the key to consistent, pain-free weight loss and is especially important when you want to get really lean (5 to 7% body fat).

So let's start at the beginning. What the hell does metabolism even mean?

The dictionary defines *metabolism* as "the chemical processes that occur within a living organism in order to maintain life."

Two kinds of metabolism are often distinguished: constructive metabolism, or *anabolism*, which is the synthesis of the proteins, carbohydrates, and fats that form tissue and store energy; and destructive metabolism, or *catabolism*, which is the breakdown of complex substances and the consequent production of energy and waste matter.

In short, when we speak of the metabolism, we speak of the body's ability to use various chemical processes to produce, maintain, and break down various substances and to make energy available for cells to use.

As you can imagine, this is an incredibly complex subject, as it encompasses the entire set of processes that sustain life, so let's hone in on the aspect of it most relevant to this chapter: metabolic speed.

What does it mean to have a "slow" or "fast" metabolism? Well, such distinctions refer to what is known as the body's *metabolic rate*, which is simply the amount of energy the body uses to perform the many functions involved in metabolism.

Basal metabolic rate (BMR) excludes physical activity, and we often measure it in terms of calories. The faster one's metabolism is, the more energy the body burns in performing the many tasks related to staying alive. The slower it is, the less energy it burns performing these tasks.

In a funny sense, a slower metabolism is actually more "efficient" than a faster one because it requires less energy to maintain life. (This doesn't mean a slow metabolism is *good*.)

Now, the body's metabolic rate is influenced by various factors such as age, fat mass, fat-free mass, and thyroid hormone circulation, but some people naturally just burn more energy than others.[48]

For instance, one study reported basal metabolic rates from as low as 1,027 calories per day to as high as 2,499 calories per day, with a mean BMR of 1,500 calories per day.[49] Much of this variance was due to different levels of fat-free mass and fat mass, age, and experimental error, but a significant portion (about 27%) of the variance was unexplained.

Another study demonstrated that basal metabolic rates can vary between people with nearly identical levels of lean mass and fat mass.[50] Researchers found that despite their subjects all having comparable body compositions, the top 5% BMRs metabolized energy about 30% faster than the lowest 5%.

So, that's what the metabolism is and how it works. Let's now relate it to weight loss.

The vast majority of your body's energy demands come from the metabolism. For instance, a 180-pound man with 10% body fat and a healthy metabolism has a basal metabolic rate of about 2,000 calories per day. Through regular exercise and other activity, total daily energy expenditure (TDEE) could increase to about 2,800 calories per day.

As we can see, about 70% of an in-shape, active man's TDEE still comes from the metabolism.

This is why preserving metabolic health is so important when it comes to weight loss. When you reduce your calorie intake to induce weight loss, you're mainly counting on your metabolism to keep humming along, pulling from fat stores. Sure, you use exercise to increase overall energy demands and thus fat loss, but your metabolism is a major player in the game.

The slower your metabolism is, the less food you'll have to eat and the more exercise you'll have to do to lose weight effectively. And when you're trying to get really lean, it can become grueling and very unhealthy.

On the other hand, the faster your metabolism is, the more you'll be able to eat and the less you'll have to exercise to lose weight (in particular, the less cardio you'll have to do, which helps you maintain lean mass).

Most people know that losing weight requires eating less food than they're currently eating and moving more, and most people want to lose weight as quickly as possible.

So what do many people do? Well, they dramatically reduce calorie intake and dramatically increase energy output (through many hours of exercise each week). And while this approach will induce weight loss for a bit, it will ultimately fail. Why?

Because your metabolism adapts to the amount of energy you feed your body. Its goal is to balance energy intake with output: to maintain homeostasis.

When you restrict your calories and feed your body less energy than it burns, your metabolism naturally begins slowing down (burning less energy). The more you restrict your calories, the faster and greater the down-regulation.[51][52]

The opposite is true as well, by the way. As you feed your body more, your metabolism will naturally speed up (burn more energy).[53]

Now, when someone dramatically decreases calorie intake and his metabolism finally slows down enough to match intake with output, weight loss stalls. This is usually met with further calorie reduction or more exercise, which only results in more metabolic slowdown, and thus a vicious cycle begins.

In most cases, the dieter finally can't take the misery anymore and goes in the other direction, dramatically increasing calorie intake (binging and gorging on everything in sight for days or weeks). This, in turn, has been shown to result in rapid fat storage, often beyond the pre-diet body fat levels (people end up fatter than when they started dieting in the first place).[54]

What's going on here is very simple: these people have systematically crashed their metabolic rates and then overloaded their bodies with way more calories than they needed, and the body's response to this is to store much of the excess energy as fat.

Ultimately, what happens is the person winds up fatter and with a slower metabolism than when he started. If he repeats this cycle a few times, he can find himself in a bad place metabolically: eating very little food to maintain a high body fat percentage.

This process of dramatically and chronically slowing down the metabolic rate is often referred to as metabolic damage, and fortunately, it can be resolved.

Your metabolic health is going to determine how effectively you can lose weight, so here's the bottom line: if you want smooth and consistent weight loss, you want your metabolism to be running quickly before you start.

As the metabolism adapts to food intake, you want your weight to be stable with a high number of daily calories before you start restricting them for weight loss purposes and especially before you undertake the journey to shredded body fat levels.

Ideally, you should be eating at least your TDEE without gaining weight before you start a weight loss routine (If you're not sure how to calculate this, we'll go over it soon).

If you're not currently there—that is, if you're eating quite a bit less than your TDEE and your weight is not moving down—you need to improve your metabolism before you attempt to get really lean.

Fortunately, this is easy to do if you remain patient. Here's how you do it:

1. Engage in heavy resistance training (ideally, weightlifting) 3 to 5 times per week

This has two big benefits for your metabolic rate: it speeds it up in the short term, burning a significant number of post-workout calories; and it builds muscle, which speeds up your metabolic rate in the long term.[55][56]

The program in this book is perfect for increasing metabolic speed.

2. Eat plenty of protein

A high-protein diet is important because it will promote muscle growth, which is what we want to achieve with step #1.

I recommend that you eat 1 gram of protein per pound of body weight when you're working on speeding up your metabolism.

3. Eat a moderate amount of dietary fat

While I'm generally not a fan of high-fat dieting for athletes, I do recommend eating a fair amount of dietary fat every day when working to improve your metabolic health.

Dietary fat boosts testosterone production (albeit slightly), which in turn speeds up metabolic rate. It's a relatively minor point, but every little bit helps.[57][58]

I recommend that you get 25 to 30% of your daily calories from dietary fat when you're working on speeding up your metabolism.

4. Slowly increase your calories each week until you've reached your target intake (your TDEE)

Instead of dramatically increasing your calorie intake, you want to raise it slowly, allowing your metabolism to keep up and match output with intake (resulting in little to no fat storage).

In the bodybuilding world, this is known as "reverse dieting," and it's a very effective way to speed up your metabolism. Here's how it works:

Week 1:

Increase your daily calorie intake by 100 by adding 25 grams of carbs to your meal plan.

If you are eating 1,800 calories per day, then you will want to eat 1,900 per day for the next 5 to 7 days.

Week 2:

Increase your daily calorie intake by 100 by adding 25 grams of carbs to your meal plan.

Same deal as the last. In keeping with the example, your intake would now go up to 2,000 calories per day for 5 to 7 days.

Week 3:

Increase your daily calorie intake by about 100 by adding 10 grams of fat to your meal plan.

Now adjust your fat intake to keep it around 30% of your total daily calories.

Week 4 and Beyond:

Increase your daily calorie intake by 100 by alternating between increasing carbohydrate and fat intake.

You continue this way, increasing daily carbohydrate intake by 25 grams for 5 to 7 days, followed by another carbohydrate intake increase (25 grams more for 5 to 7 days), followed by a fat intake increase (10 grams more for 5 to 7 days), until you've reached your TDEE for your *current* weight.

This last point is minor but worth addressing. As you do this, your weight will go up. Don't worry, you aren't gaining a bunch of fat; your muscles are simply filling up with glycogen and water.

When your metabolism is healthy—when you're able to eat plenty of food every day without storing fat—weight loss, and even getting really lean, is quite straightforward. You can get the job done with a mild calorie deficit and 4 to 6 hours of exercise per week.

Yes, your metabolism will slow down, but not by much. This approach will give you at least a good 2- to 3-month window for steady, consistent fat loss.

And if, over time, your metabolism slows down too much but you haven't hit your body fat percentage goal yet, you simply take the above steps to speed your metabolism back up and then move back to weight loss.

So, now that we know where we want our metabolic speed to be before attempting to get really lean, let's look at some nutrition and exercise strategies for getting shredded.

17

HOW TO GET SHREDDED WITHOUT FRYING YOUR MUSCLES OR YOUR SANITY

GETTING REALLY LEAN IS THE BODYBUILDING equivalent of getting rich and feeling you've "arrived."

It's the first big payoff for years of hard work, and it's when people start to notice your physique. You're no longer known as just the "big guy"—you're now the "shredded guy."

What does it take to get there? Why do single-digit body fat percentages elude so many?

If you're like most guys, you've probably found or will find that getting to the range of 10% body fat is fairly straightforward and comfortable. You restrict your calories, stick to your workout routine, and things just roll along smoothly.

Getting below, however, can be quite a grind if you do it wrong.

Your strength can nosedive, you can lose a considerable amount of visual size, you can struggle with hunger and cravings, and more. In short, you can be completely miserable.

Fortunately, it doesn't have to be this way. You can get shredded without turning into a scrawny weakling and without fantasizing about what types of felonies you would commit for some carbs.

This chapter will provide you with a variety of tools and strategies that you will be able to use to get super lean while maintaining as much size, strength, and sanity as possible.

So, let's start with the heart of the issue. Why does it get harder and harder to get leaner and leaner, and why does getting rid of the last bit of ab and lower back fat seem almost impossible?

The answer has to do with what is commonly referred to as stubborn fat.

THE SCIENCE OF STUBBORN FAT

To understand why it's so damn hard to get shredded, you need to understand how and why fat is stored and mobilized.

When you eat food, your body breaks it down into various substances, one of which is glucose, or blood sugar.

Your body also releases the hormone insulin, which tells your liver, muscles, and fat tissue to take the glucose from the blood and store it.

Your liver and muscles store the glucose as a substance known as glycogen, and your fat cells store it as a substance known as triglycerides.

The storage of glycogen expands the size of the muscle cells, and the storage of triglycerides expands the fat cells, which in turn expands your waistline.

When you're in this "fed" state, no fat burning occurs. Your body uses the glucose in the blood for all its energy needs and stores the excess. Depending on how much you eat, this state can last for several hours.[59][60]

But, as the nutrients eaten are absorbed, insulin levels decline, and the body senses that its post-meal energy is running out. It then shifts toward burning fat stores to meet its energy needs. Day after day, it juggles these states of storing nutrients you eat and burning its stores when the temporary supplies run out.

To burn, or mobilize, fat, your body produces chemicals known as catecholamines. The catecholamines travel through your blood and attach to receptors on fat cells, which triggers the release of the energy stored within the cells so you can burn it off.

Fat cells have two types of receptors for catecholamines: alpha-2 and beta-2 receptors. To keep this simple, beta-2 receptors speed up fat mobilization, whereas alpha-2 receptors hinder it.[61][62]

So, here's the big difference between regular and stubborn fat: fat that is easy to lose has more beta-2 receptors than alpha-2, and fat that is hard to lose has more alpha-2 receptors than beta-2. This ratio of alpha-2 and beta-2 receptors in individual fat cells determines how easy or hard it is to mobilize the energy stored inside.

Let's now tie this back into the overall subject at hand.

As you get leaner, you have less and less regular and more and more stubborn fat on your body. In my experience, a large amount of the fat you lose going from the 9% range to the 6% range is stubborn fat.

This is why efficiently dieting from 10% down to 6% is slower and trickier (it requires more attention to caloric intake, more caloric adjustments, and usually supplementation) than dieting from 15% down to 10%.

There's another aspect of this to consider: *time.*

A big mistake many guys make when cutting is they simply drag it out too long. There are several downsides to this.

The longer you remain in a calorie deficit, even when it's mild, the more your metabolism slows down, the more muscle you lose, the more your body becomes stressed,[63] and the more your anabolic hormones decrease.[64 65 66]

Furthermore, there's the psychological aspect as well. The longer you have to diet, the more likely you are to give up.

In my opinion, the goal when cutting should be to achieve the desired body fat percentage as quickly as possible while sacrificing little to no muscle or strength.

Sound like a pipe dream? Well, it's not—anyone, no matter his genetics, can do it.

With that, let's now begin looking at the practical side of this chapter: exercise, nutrition, and supplementation strategies that will make the journey to 6 or 7% as painless as possible.

Remember that you should follow these strategies in addition to maintaining a mild daily or weekly calorie deficit (about 20%), as this is the basis of all healthy weight loss. If you're not sure how to do this, then I recommend you read *BLS.*

NUTRITION STRATEGIES FOR GETTING SHREDDED

I have good news: it's likely that you won't need to do anything particularly special nutritionally to get shredded.

Although we'll talk about them later, you probably won't have to follow unorthodox dietary protocols like intermittent fasting or carb cycling, and you won't have to severely restrict the types of foods you eat or starve yourself.

The biggest part of getting shredded is just patience.

Once you get below 10% body fat, you shouldn't expect to lose more than 0.5 to 1 pound of fat per week. You might be able to lose around 1 pound per week at 10%, but you'll find yourself losing 0.5 pounds per week at 8%.

To put things into perspective, when I do everything you're learning in this chapter, it takes me about 6 to 8 weeks to go from 9% down to 6% body fat. It takes about the same amount of time to go from 15% down to 10%.

So, if you're currently above 10%, don't set unreal expectations for yourself by assuming that you will get absolutely ripped in a couple of months without burning up a bunch of muscle. It doesn't work like that.

However, the nice thing about dieting properly is that it isn't grueling, and with a proper reverse diet, it's quite easy to maintain a ripped physique for months at a time, or even year-round.

Now, let's get to the nutrition and supplementation strategies.

BE METICULOUS WITH YOUR CALORIC INTAKE

The reality is you just don't have much wiggle room with your numbers as you get leaner and leaner: your metabolism is slowing down, and overeating has a much more noticeable effect on your progress.

Don't add little snacks because you're hungry; use the hunger control strategies outlined in the next chapter instead. Don't go for a few more bites every meal; those calories can add up quickly. Don't get into the habit of trying to make too many on-the-fly adjustments to your meal plan; this tends to lead to overeating.

This last point warrants more discussion. In terms of tracking your intake, you have two options:

1. Create a meal plan that you follow every day.

2. Make food choices on the fly using an application like MyFitnessPal to count calories/macros.

I much prefer creating a meal plan for a few reasons:

1. It helps me time and size my meals optimally.

    By optimally, I mean best for my preferences and body. I like eating every few hours with more or less the same number of calories in each meal. This keeps me from getting overly hungry. When you track on the fly, however, you can easily fall prey to the tendency to want to just keep eating at each meal. Then, come dinnertime, you can find yourself with few calories left, which means you get to go hungry for the rest of the night.

2. It helps me get the most enjoyment out of my calories.

    When I'm cutting, I like to stick to relatively low-calorie foods that taste good simply because I get to eat more of them. This makes dieting more enjoyable (the more tasty food you get to eat, the better).

    Some foods are just too calorie-dense for me to want to eat because it'll mean I have to skimp on later meals. By planning my meals ahead of time, I can give some thought as to how to best eat my calories. If you're tracking on the fly, it's easier to "waste" calories in meals that you could've saved for later and enjoyed more.

3. I don't want to have to think about what I'm going to eat next or worry about how many calories I have left.

    I have an incredibly busy schedule, and I don't want to bother with trying to decide what to eat and when. I like to have it worked out and prepared beforehand, so I can just quickly enjoy the meal and move on with my day.

SIMPLIFY YOUR MEAL PLAN

This isn't entirely necessary, but it definitely helps you ensure you're not accidentally eating more than you should.

Now, I'm not saying you should eat nothing but boiled chicken, baked sweet potatoes, and steamed broccoli, but you would be smart to avoid meals that you can't fully account for in terms of calories. Eating out can be a huge problem, as can homemade meals that aren't controlled in terms of portion size and macronutrients.

What I like to do is stick to relatively simple foods that are dense in micronutrients, like the following:

- Avocados

- Greens (chard, collard greens, kale, mustard greens, spinach)

- Bell peppers

- Brussels sprouts

- Mushrooms

- Baked potatoes

- Sweet potatoes

- Berries

- Low-fat Greek yogurt

- Eggs

- Seeds (flax, pumpkin, sesame, and sunflower)

- Beans (garbanzo, kidney, navy, pinto)

- Lentils, peas

- Almonds, cashews, peanuts

- Barley, oats, quinoa, brown rice

- Salmon, halibut, cod, scallops, shrimp, tuna

- Lean beef, lamb, venison

- Chicken, turkey

I will just get creative with how I prepare them, relying on recipes from my cookbooks *The Shredded Chef* and *Eat Green Get Lean*, or keeping it really simple with various types of zero-calorie spices as well as low-calorie sauces like mustards, salsa, and hot sauces.

Furthermore, different types of cooking methods can turn an otherwise boring meal into something incredibly tasty. I'm hot on one-pot cooking these days because it not only delivers some outstanding food, but it also requires no special culinary skills and minimal prep and cleanup (one pot!).

So, to wrap up this point, I recommend sticking to foods you like; just reduce the margin for error in terms of caloric intake by simplifying your meal plan. Use a website like CalorieKing to research the macronutrient profiles of various foods, and piece your meal plan together meal by meal.

SCHEDULE YOUR MEALS FOR SUCCESS

I have good news for you:

You don't have to eat meals on any set schedule to lose weight or build muscle efficiently. A proper meal schedule is one that fits your schedule.

You see, meal frequency has little relevance on actual results. You can eat 3 meals per day or 9 and achieve the same thing if you're doing everything else right in terms of your calorie intake, macronutrient ratios, and exercise regimen.

That said, unless you definitely prefer fewer meals, or must eat fewer due to your schedule/lifestyle, I actually do recommend you plan to eat every 3 – 4 hours. Why? Because in my experience, most people find this easiest in terms of overall enjoyment, staving off hunger when cutting and getting in enough food when bulking.

In terms of meal timing, there are only two meals I recommend you "time":

1. Unless you're training fasted, have 30 grams of protein and 30 – 50 grams of carbohydrate before your weightlifting. This will not only give you a nice boost of energy for your workouts, it can help you build more muscle over time.[67] You don't necessarily need food before cardio, but 20 grams of protein isn't a bad idea as it will help minimize muscle damage.

2. Have 30 – 50 grams of protein and about 30% of your daily carbs in your post-workout meal. This will help your body replenish depleted glycogen stores and can also help you build more muscle over time.[68][69]

That's it. The rest of your meals can be timed however you please, so just work it around your preferences and schedule. Again, you will probably find a smaller meal every few hours most enjoyable, but feel free to experiment.

You can also play with when you start eating for the day. If you like eating breakfast, eat one. If you don't, and would prefer to wait until lunch before you start eating, you can do that too. Sometimes skipping that first meal (which will not "make you fat," like some people claim) helps with overall compliance as it allows you to eat larger meals and still stick to your numbers.[70]

REDUCE YOUR CALORIES AS YOU GET LEANER

As you know, when you restrict your calories to lose fat, your metabolism naturally slows down. You can minimize this with proper nutrition and regular exercise, but it's just a fact of dieting.[71]

For this reason, you will find that your weight loss will stall after a certain period at a given caloric intake. The way through this plateau is to either increase activity or reduce calories.

I like to increase activity up to lifting 5 times per week and doing cardio 4 times per week (about 30 minutes of HIIT per session), but going beyond that causes significant reductions in strength, which indicates the onset of overtraining. At that point, I begin reducing calories.

You don't want to make large reductions, however. As you know, a severe calorie deficit leads to all kinds of trouble.

The best way to go about it is to reduce your daily intake by 100 calories (pull from carbs—keep your protein high and your fats no lower than 0.2 grams per pound of body weight) for 7 to 10 days and see whether that does it.

If you lose weight in those 7 to 10 days, keep your caloric intake at this level and see whether you can lose more over the next 7 to 10 days. If you don't lose weight from the initial reduction, drop your intake by another 100 calories and see if that does it.

Simply work your calories down in this way, gradually reducing them along with your body fat.

When you should start reducing intake depends on your body. You start with the simple weight-loss formula laid out in *BLS* (1.2 grams of protein per pound of body weight; 1 gram of carbohydrate per pound; and .2 grams of fat per pound) and stay there until you don't lose any weight for 7 to 10 days. You then reduce intake by 100 calories per day, re-evaluate, etc.

There's a point where you want to stop reducing calories as well, regardless of whether you've reached your body fat goal, as further reductions can lead to the metabolic damage we've already talked about.

I stop reducing my calories when my intake reaches my BMR for my current weight (not my starting weight) to preserve metabolic health and muscle.

You can calculate your BMR by using the Katch McArdle formula. If you're not familiar with this formula, here's how it works:

$$BMR = 370 + (21.6 * LBM)$$

LBM refers to lean body mass in kilograms, and you calculate lean body mass by subtracting your body fat weight from your total body weight (it's the weight of everything but your body fat).

Here's how you calculate LBM:

$$LBM = (1 – BF\%) * total\ body\ weight$$

For instance, I'm currently 192 pounds at about 7% body fat, so my LBM is calculated like this:

$$1 – 0.07 = 0.93$$
$$0.93 * 192 = 178\ pounds\ (LBM)$$

There are 2.2 pounds in each kilogram, so here is the formula to calculate my BMR:

$$178 / 2.2 = 81\ kg$$
$$370 + (21.6 * 81) = 2,100\ calories\ per\ day$$

Before we move on, let's see how this all works in the real world, using my last cut from 9% down to 6% body fat as an example.

I started at 194 pounds, and I reduced my daily caloric intake to 2,400 per day. That brought about 8 pounds of weight loss over the course of 4 weeks (I lost several pounds of water weight in the first 2 weeks), at which point my weight loss stalled and I had to drop to 2,300 per day.

Over the course of the next 3 to 4 weeks, I gradually reduced to 2,000 calories per day, which was my approximate BMR for my final weight of 184 pounds, as calculated with the Katch McArdle formula.

I stayed at 2,000 calories per day for another 2 weeks to squeeze out the last bits of fat loss and then began increasing caloric intake. I subsequently lost a bit more weight as a result of reducing cortisol levels, which in turn reduced water retention.

My final weight was 182 pounds, somewhere around 5 to 6% body fat:

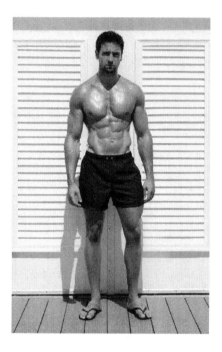

This is the best way to go about reducing calorie intake to ensure you continue losing fat without burning up too much muscle.

Now, it can happen that your intake reaches your BMR, but you haven't yet reached your desired body fat percentage. This is okay.

The solution isn't to increase training frequency or further reduce calories. Stay at your BMR intake until weight loss stops, and then begin reverse dieting to speed up your metabolism. You will gain minimal body fat in this period, if any at all.

Once you've completed your reverse diet (you're able to eat your

TDEE without gaining weight), you can begin cutting again and should have plenty of time to now reach your desired look.

REFEED, DON'T CHEAT

As you get leaner, your cheating needs to serve a purpose beyond enjoying yourself. Instead of hitting a restaurant and going full Jabba, you need to schedule refeeds.

(If you don't remember this from *BLS*, a refeed is a day where in you dramatically increase carb and reduce fat intake, resulting in a moderate increase in caloric intake.)

The reason for increasing both caloric and carbohydrate intake goes beyond the psychological boost, which helps keep you happy and motivated and more likely to stay the course. There are very important physiological reasons as well.

The physical reasons relate to a hormone called *leptin*, which regulates hunger, your metabolic rate, appetite, motivation, and libido; it also serves other functions in your body.[72][73][74]

When you're in a caloric deficit and lose body fat, your leptin levels drop and can become chronically low.[75] This, in turn, causes your metabolic rate to slow down, your appetite to increase, your motivation to wane, and your mood to sour.

When you give your body more energy (calories) than it needs, leptin levels rise, which can then have positive effects on fat oxidation, thyroid activity, mood, and even testosterone levels.[76][77][78][79]

So if it's an increase in leptin levels that you want, how do you best achieve it?

You refeed, because eating carbohydrates is the most effective way to spike leptin levels.[80] Protein can also raise leptin levels as well as increase leptin sensitivity (the more sensitive your body is to leptin, the better it responds to its signals).[81] However, dietary fats aren't very effective at increasing leptin levels, and alcohol inhibits it.[82][83]

A proper refeed is very simple. Over the course of ONE day, you...

- Reduce protein intake to 0.8 grams per pound of body weight.

- Increase carb intake to 2 grams per pound of body weight.

- Reduce fat intake to 0.1 to 0.15 grams per pound of body

weight.

How often you should refeed depends partially on your body, but most people don't need to do it more than once every 5 to 7 days, which is my general recommendation.

I also recommend that you do it in the middle of your training week. The increase in carbs will give you a nice boost of strength in the gym. (I like to do it before back or legs to help with deadlifting or squatting.)

THE DEAL WITH LOW-CARB DIETING

The hysterical crusade against carbohydrates has reached a frantic pitch.

From the scientifically bankrupt theories of guys like Gary Taubes to the trendy low-carb diets like Paleo, Zone, Dukan, and so forth, the carbohydrate is now the victim of the same level of persecution that saturated fat endured for decades.

Well, we've come to learn that saturated fats aren't the evil heart killers they were made out to be (excluding the processed form known as trans fat, which is known to increase risk of heart disease, among other issues).[84] [85]

If we're to believe the leaders of the Carbohydrate Inquisition, this molecule will blow up our blood sugar levels, break our metabolism, force us to be fat, give us diabetes and many other diseases, and, well, just generally turn us into hungry, horrible people.

If we just ditch the diabolical carbohydrate, "experts" claim we will melt fat away and keep it off without having to count pesky calories, build an invincible immune system, live forever, and maybe even develop superpowers. And we'll be part of the cool crowd to boot.

So, is this culture war justified? Does it have a basis in science?

CARBOHYDRATES, INSULIN LEVELS, AND WEIGHT GAIN

Much of the controversy revolves around carbohydrates' relationship with the hormone *insulin*.

As the claims go, insulin makes you fat, and carbohydrates spike insulin, thus, carbohydrates make you fat. Sounds so simple, right? Well, yeah, the story is simple…but it's false.

While yes, it's true that insulin's job is to pull glucose out of the blood and store excess as fat, it's also responsible for driving amino acids into our muscles for protein synthesis and clearing dietary fats out of the blood as well (which are stored as body fat more efficiently than carbohydrates, I might add).[86] On top of all that, insulin has a mild anti-catabolic effect (meaning it helps preserve your muscle).[87]

And while it's also true that eating carbohydrates increases insulin levels in your blood, many common sources of protein (such as eggs, cheese, beef, and fish) cause the same types of insulin responses.[88]

Some people claim that because your body generally produces more insulin when you eat carbohydrates, this leads to more fat storage. They're wrong: research has shown that the amount of insulin your body produces in response to eating food (or insulin response, as it's called) doesn't affect the amount of fat stored.[89]

So, in short, insulin is your friend, not a part of a conspiracy between your pancreas and fat cells to ruin your self-image.

That's one strike against the "carbs make you fat" camp. Let's now look directly at carbohydrate intake and fat loss.

DIET COMPOSITION AND REAL-WORLD WEIGHT LOSS

Many low-carb gurus will claim that you can lose weight much more quickly if you consume very few carbs every day. Some people even believe they can only lose weight if they cut their carbs to nil.

The problem with this advice and belief is they fly in the face of both basic physiology and scientific findings and mask the most common weight-loss roadblocks: eating too much and moving too little.

A simple review of scientific literature shows that diet composition has no effect on long-term weight loss.

For example, let's first look at a study conducted by researchers at the University of Pennsylvania.[90] Researchers assigned 63 obese adults to either a low-carbohydrate, high-protein, high-fat diet (20 grams of carbohydrate per day, gradually increased until target weight was achieved) or a conventional diet of 60% of calories from carbohydrates, 25% from fats, and 15% from protein.

The result: the low-carbohydrate group lost more weight in the first 3 months, but the difference at 12 months wasn't significant.

The 3-month result isn't surprising, considering the fact that reducing carbohydrate intake decreases the amount of glycogen we store in our liver and muscles, which in turn decreases total body water retention.[91][92] This, of course, causes a rapid drop in weight that has nothing to do with burning fat (and anyone who has reduced carbohydrate intake as a means of cutting calories for weight loss has experienced this).

Researchers from Harvard University published a study in 2009 on the effects of diet composition and weight loss.[93] The researchers assigned 811 overweight adults to one of three diets, which consisted of the following percentages of fat, protein, and carbs: 20% F, 15% P, and 65% C; 40% F, 15% P, and 45% C; and 40% F, 25% P, and 35% C.

After 6 months of dieting, participants had lost and average of 6 kilograms. They began to regain weight after 12 months, and by 2 years, weight loss averaged out to 4 kilograms, with no meaningful differences between low-protein or high-protein, low-fat or high-fat, and low-carb or high-carb groups.

A study published by researchers at Arizona State University found that an 8-week high-carbohydrate, low-fat, low-protein diet and a low-carbohydrate, low-fat, high-protein diet were equally effective in terms of weight loss.[94]

So, the conclusion we can derive is brutally simple and clear: as long as you keep yourself in a caloric deficit, you'll lose weight regardless of the dietary protocol you follow.[95]

WHEN LOW-CARB—OR HIGH-CARB—CAN BE BETTER

Despite the body of evidence presented above, practical experience in coaching hundreds of people has taught me that some people tend to just do better on high-carb or low-carb diets, and some do fine with either.

For instance, some people—like me—do very well with high-carbohydrate diets. They can lose weight very easily, feel energized all day without any crashes, and are able to maintain considerable strength in the gym. Others don't do well with a high-carb approach. Weight loss is slower than optimal; it makes them very hungry, which leads to overeating; and it comes with frustrating energy highs and lows.

It goes the other way too. Some people don't do well with low-carb, high-fat diets (me, again). They feel lethargic and mentally clouded, lose a ton of strength, and have trouble getting lean. Others thrive on it, having plenty of energy and a general sense of well-being.

What gives?

Well, while feeling like crap makes you more likely to overeat or mess up your diet in other ways and give less than 100% in your workouts, there's more at work here.

Research has shown that some people's bodies deal better with large amounts of dietary fat than others, responding with positive metabolic changes like an increase in resting energy expenditure and fat oxidation to maintain energy balance and better appetite control.[96][97][98] Some people's bodies respond negatively to high amounts of dietary fat, however, and are more likely to store it as body fat. Such research sheds some light on why some people respond so well or poorly to low-carb, high-fat diets. A ketogenic diet (very low-carbohydrate intake) can be a disaster for some and a godsend for others.

The above also relates to research on how insulin sensitivity and insulin response affect diet effectiveness.[99] (Remember that insulin sensitivity refers to how responsive your cells are to insulin's signals, and insulin response—or insulin secretion—refers to how much insulin is secreted into your blood in response to food eaten.)

Research has shown that weight loss efforts aren't improved or impaired by insulin sensitivity levels per se.[100] However, when we move away from a balance of nutrients and use high-carb, low-fat, or low-carb, high-fat diets in conjunction with different levels of insulin sensitivity and insulin response, things change.

For instance, a study conducted by the Tufts-New England Medical Center found that a low-glycemic load diet helped overweight adults with high insulin secretion lose more weight, but it did not have the same effect on overweight adults with low insulin secretion.[101]

A study conducted by researchers at the University of Colorado demonstrated that obese women who were insulin sensitive lost significantly more weight on a high-carb, low-fat diet than a low-carb, high-fat diet (average weight loss of 13.5% vs. 6.8% of body weight, respectively); those who were insulin resistant lost significantly more weight on a low-carb, high-fat diet than a high-carb, low-fat diet (average weight loss of 13.4% vs. 8.5% of body weight, respectively).[102]

What we can take away from my anecdotal observations and these studies is if you have good insulin sensitivity and low insulin secretion (good insulin response), you'll probably do better on a high-carb, low-fat diet. On the other hand, if you have poor insulin sensitivity (insulin resistance) and high secretion (poor insulin response), you'll probably do better on a low-carb, high-fat diet.

SO, WHICH APPROACH, THEN? HIGH-CARB OR LOW-CARB?

Unfortunately, it's not easy to tell whether you're a high-carb or low-carb body type, but it's fairly easy to take an educated guess regarding insulin resistance, sensitivity, and response.

After eating a high-carb meal, signs of good insulin sensitivity and response are pumped muscles that feel "full," mental alertness, stable energy levels (no crash), and satiety. Signs of insulin resistance and poor insulin response are bloat, gassiness, mental fogginess, an inability to focus, sleepiness, and hunger soon after eating.

In my experience, people with suboptimal insulin sensitivity and response do best with a low-carb approach once they get below 10%. And to quantify low-carb, anything below 0.5 grams of carbs per pound of body weight per day fits the bill.

But if your insulin response and sensitivity are good, you shouldn't have to drastically reduce carbs to get shredded. You will have to walk them down as discussed earlier, but I've never had to go lower than 0.8 grams per pound of body weight per day.

EXERCISE STRATEGIES FOR GETTING SHREDDED

Let's break exercise down into two categories: weightlifting and cardio.

When you're cutting, you lift weights primarily to burn calories and preserve muscle and strength, and you do cardio primarily to burn calories.

Many "gurus" recommend that you follow a high-rep, low-weight routine to help shred up, but this is idiotic and the complete opposite of what you want to do.

You see, when you restrict your calories intake for fat loss, it reduces anabolic hormone levels and suppresses protein synthesis rates.[103] [104] That is, your body is primed for muscle loss when you're dieting to lose fat, and you want to take measures to counteract this. By focusing exclusively on muscle endurance (higher rep ranges), however, you'll be setting yourself up for rapid strength loss, with the potential for significant muscle loss as well.

Instead, you want to focus on lifting heavy weights and try to actually progress in your strength while you're cutting. I've found that I usually progress for the first 3 – 4 weeks and then stall, at which point my goal is to maintain as much of that strength as possible.

That said, when you're cutting, I recommend you drop the Sarcoplasmic Hypertrophy Sets from the *Beyond Bigger Leaner Stronger* workouts for two reasons: it reduces the amount of stress on the body, thus preventing overtraining, and higher rep work is really draining when you're in a calorie deficit.

Now let's talk about some specific exercise strategies that will help you get shredded.

TRAINING FREQUENCY

The more you exercise, the more fat you burn, but if you push things too hard, you can quickly find yourself bloated and burned out.

You see, just being in a calorie deficit raises cortisol levels and intense exercise—both lifting and cardio—further stresses the body.[105]

The proper training frequency is one that provides maximum fat loss while keeping stress levels relatively low and under control.

There are many opinions as to what this means in actual hours spent in the gym, however.

On one end of the spectrum are the "no pain, no gain" types who want to spend 10+ hours per week exercising, and on the other end are the conservative types who believe you should dramatically reduce training frequency while cutting to avoid overstressing the body.

The reality is there is no one-size-fits-all answer to optimal training frequency, as some people's bodies deal with stress better than others. But in my experience, both with my body and with the hundreds of people I've worked with, it's harder to reach this point of overtraining than some experts believe. Generally speaking, readers on my programs have absolutely no issues lifting 5 times per week and doing cardio 3 to 4 times per week while cutting—a total of about 5 to 7 hours of exercise per week. I've yet to meet someone who had to scale back his lifting and cardio back to 2 or 3 times per week.

This is likely due to a combination of factors: proper training volume (the workouts aren't long, grueling bloodbaths), proper nutrition (mild calorie deficit, good macronutrient ratios, plenty of micronutrient-dense foods), relatively short (about 25 minutes) HIIT cardio sessions, proper rest, and more.

If you were to mess with any of those factors—make the workouts too long or too intense, make the calorie deficit too severe, replace nutritious foods with junk, or work out too much and/or sleep too little—it's likely that people would run into trouble.

So, that's why I recommend a moderately high training frequency when you want to get lean: specifically, lifting 5 times per week and doing cardio 3 to 4 times per week.

We want to use the exercise to drive the fat loss, and if you keep in mind the basics that you learned in *BLS*, it's unlikely that you'll burn out.

DO HIGH-INTENSITY INTERVAL CARDIO

This is a point I talk about in *BLS*, but I want to reiterate it here because it's especially useful when you want to get super lean and preserve muscle.

Studies such as those conducted by researchers at Laval University, East Tennessee State University, Baylor College of Medicine, and the University of New South Wales have shown that shorter, high-intensity cardio sessions result in greater fat loss over time than longer, low-intensity sessions.[106 107 108 109]

A study conducted by researchers at the University of Western Ontario gives us insight into how much more effective it is. Researchers had 10 men and 10 women train 3 times per week, with one group doing 4 to 6 30-second treadmill sprints (with 4 to 6 minutes of rest in between each), and the other group doing 30 to 60 minutes of steady-state cardio (running on the treadmill at the magical fat loss zone of

65% VO2 max).[110]

The results: After 6 weeks of training, the subjects doing the intervals had lost more fat. Yes, 4 to 6 30-second sprints burn more fat than 60 minutes of incline treadmill walking.

Although the exact mechanisms of how high-intensity cardio trumps steady-state cardio aren't fully understood yet, scientists have isolated quite a few of the factors:

- Increased resting metabolic rate for more than 24 hours after exercise

- Improved insulin sensitivity in the muscles

- Higher levels of fat oxidation in the muscles

- Significant spikes in growth hormone levels (which aid in fat loss) and catecholamine levels (the chemicals your body produces that help burn fat)

- Post-exercise appetite suppression[111]

The bottom line is that high-intensity interval training (HIIT) burns more fat in less time than steady-state cardio.

And what about muscle preservation?

Well, research has shown that the longer your cardio sessions are, the more they impair strength and hypertrophy.[112] That is, the shorter your cardio sessions are, the more muscle you preserve. Thus, keeping your cardio sessions short is important when we're talking about preserving your muscle.

Furthermore, research has also shown that endurance training directly interferes with strength and hypertrophy (muscle growth) progress.[113] This is why I'm stingy with my cardio. I want to do just enough to keep the fat loss going, but no more.

Well, only HIIT allows you to both keep the duration and frequency of your cardio sessions short while still deriving significant benefits from the exercise.

Now, you might be wondering what the best forms of HIIT are. Well, my favorite HIIT routine is cycling (recumbent cycling, to be specific), and here's why: it's not only convenient that I can bring my iPad and read or watch a show or movie while doing my cardio, but it also turns out that cycling itself has special benefits for us weightlifters.

These benefits were demonstrated in a particularly interesting study conducted by researchers from Stephen F Austin State University.[114]

What researchers found is that the *type* of cardio done had a profound effect on the subjects' ability to gain strength and size in their weightlifting. The subjects who did running and walking for their cardio gained significantly less strength and size than those who cycled.

Why?

Researchers concluded that it was because cycling involves the use of more of the muscles used in hypertrophy movements (Squats, for instance) than running or walking does. That is, it more closely imitates the motions that result in hypertrophy and thus doesn't impair hypertrophy.

Therefore, I recommend cycling for your HIIT if you have access to a bike. If you don't, rowing is also a good method for the same reasons (it imitates upper body hypertrophy movements), and sprinting is as well. As you know, I recommend keeping your sessions relatively short (20 to 30 minutes).

In terms of an exact protocol, here's what you can do.

1. You start your workout with 2 to 3 minutes of low-intensity warm-up on the lowest resistance (if you're using a machine with resistance).

2. You then up the resistance (if applicable) and pedal, row, run, etc. with all-out exertion for 30 to 45 seconds.

    Really what you're looking to achieve here is a dramatic spike in your heart rate. After your first or second bout of all-out exertion, you want to see your heart rate rising to around 90% of its maximum. (And you calculate Maximum Heart Rate as follows: 205.8–[0.685 × Age].)

3. You then lower the resistance and move at a moderate pace for 60 to 90 seconds. If you're new to HIIT, you may need to extend this rest period to 2 to 4 minutes. What you want to see is a significant reduction in heart rate before starting your next high-intensity interval. I like to see

my heart rate come down to 60 to 70% of its maximum during my rest intervals.

4. You repeat this cycle of all-out and recovery intervals for 20 to 30 minutes.

5. You do a 2- to 3-minute cooldown at a low intensity.

Before we move on, I want to note that while HIIT cardio is best for maximizing fat loss, it does place more stress on the body than steady-state cardio.

If you follow my recommendations of lifting 5 times per week and doing HIIT cardio 3 to 4 times per week and begin feeling overtrained, then I recommend you replace HIIT cardio sessions with low-intensity steady-state (LISS) and see whether that helps.

Start with replacing one HIIT session with LISS and see how you feel that week. If you're still having issues, replace another and see whether that does it. Continue this until you're feeling better or all HIIT sessions are now LISS.

If you're *still* feeling overtrained, then drop cardio days altogether (one at a time). If that doesn't do it, then it's time to reverse diet for a few weeks to give your body a break and possibly to even take a Rest or Deload Week and begin cutting again once you feel better.

TRY TRAINING IN A FASTED STATE

Your body is in a fasted state when insulin is at a baseline level and your body is relying on its energy stores.

When you exercise in a fasted state, fat loss is accelerated.[115] Fasted training first thing in the morning has an added benefit, as fasting for longer than 6 hours increases your body's ability to burn fat.[116]

Weight training a fasted state is particularly effective and, as an interesting bonus, research has shown that weightlifting in a fasted state results in an improved anabolic response to a post-workout meal.[117] [118]

However, fasted training does have one significant drawback: accelerated breakdown of muscle tissue. Fortunately, preventing this is simple.[119]

You should supplement with BCAAs or 5 grams of leucine (as this amino acid directly stimulates protein synthesis) 10 to 15 minutes before training, which will suppress muscle breakdown during your workout.[120] [121]

The easiest way to train in a truly fasted state is to either lift or do your cardio after you wake up. So long as you didn't eat a massive meal before going to bed, your insulin levels will be at true baseline levels.

Once you've started eating, however, it can take anywhere from 2 to 6+ hours for your body to return to a fasted state.

One study showed that the insulin response to the ingestion of 45 grams of whey protein peaked at about 40 minutes, and these levels were sustained for about 2 hours.[122] Another study showed that the ingestion of a mixed meal containing 75 grams of carbs, 37 grams of protein, and 17 grams of fat resulted in an elevation of insulin levels for more than 5 hours (at the 5-hour mark, when researchers stopped testing, insulin levels were still double the fasting level).[123]

The significance of this is that the higher your insulin levels are, the less fat your body will burn. This is because insulin regulates lipolysis, which is the chemical process whereby the body breaks down fat cells into usable energy.[124] This is why fasted training results in more fat loss (the lower your insulin levels, the more lipolysis is possible).

What I personally do when cutting is lift early in the morning in a fasted state (I have 5 grams of leucine before training), and when I do cardio, I do it 3 to 4 hours after a light dinner (with 5 grams of leucine before this as well). This may not be enough time for my insulin levels to return to baseline, but it's probably close.

I should note that some people simply don't do well with fasted weightlifting. They have very low energy levels, and their strength takes a nosedive. If that happens to you, give it a week. If your body isn't able to adapt to it, then you should reduce the frequency (maybe lifting fasted only 1 or 2 days per week, and on days where you train smaller muscle groups like shoulders or arms) or stop altogether. Keeping your workouts intense is more important.

Another option is to do your cardio first thing in the morning (fasted) and your lifting later in the day, when the food you've eaten all day will help boost your strength and energy.

SUPPLEMENTATION STRATEGIES
FOR GETTING SHREDDED

As you know, supplementation is the least important aspect of the fitness game—proper diet and training are what builds physiques.

That said, supplementation *can* help, and even if it's not dramatic, it can be worth it in my opinion.

In the case of cutting, I've cut both with and without the supplementation routine I'm going to lay out here, and there's no question—following the routine speeds up the fat loss.

How much is hard to exactly quantify, but if I had to try, I would say that fat loss was something around 20% faster with supplementation (my cuts are always 8 to 10 weeks, so I can guess with some accuracy).

So, let's get to the supplements that can help.

CAFFEINE

Caffeine, the world's most popular drug, has more value to us fitness folks than the energy high.

It can improve strength, muscle endurance, and anaerobic performance; reverse the morning weakness experienced by many weightlifters; and, last but not least, speed up fat loss.[125] [126] [127] [128] [129]

The mechanism by which it aids weight loss is quite simple: it speeds up your body's metabolic rate by increasing the number of *catecholamines* in the blood.[130] [131]

Now, you can get your caffeine from a beverage like coffee, but interestingly enough, research has shown that the pure form you find in most pills and powders (caffeine anhydrous) is more effective for improving performance.[132]

Thus, I recommend you take caffeine pills.

If you're training fasted, take the caffeine 5 to 10 minutes before starting training. If you're not training fasted, have it 15 to 20 minutes before training.

To maximize caffeine's effectiveness, you want to prevent your body from building up too much of a tolerance.

The best way to do this is to limit intake, of course. Here's what I recommend:

1. Before training, supplement with 3 to 6 milligrams of caffeine per kilogram of body weight. If you're not sure of your caffeine sensitivity, start with 3 milligrams per kilogram and work up from there.

2. Keep your daily intake at or below 6 milligrams per kilogram of body weight. Don't have 6 milligrams per kilogram before training and then drink a couple of coffees throughout the day.

3. Do 1 or 2 low-caffeine days per week and one no-caffeine day per week. A low day should be half your normal intake, and a no day means fewer than 50 milligrams of caffeine (you can have a cup or two of tea, but no coffee, caffeine pills, etc.).

GREEN TEA EXTRACT

Green tea extract is a weight-loss supplement made from green tea leaves.

It's rich in antioxidants known as catechins, which are responsible for many of tea's health benefits and have been proven to help with weight loss.[133] [134] Research has also shown that catechins can help reduce abdominal fat, in particular.[135]

Catechins accelerate fat loss by blocking an enzyme that degrades catecholamines, which allows them to remain in your blood longer and mobilize more fat stores.[136]

Where many people go wrong with green tea extract supplementation, however, is they simply don't take enough.

If you look at the dosages proven effective in clinical studies, you'll see that 400 to 600 milligrams of catechins per day is the normal range.[137]

Ideally, you take your GTE before fasted training as research has shown that absorption is faster when pills are taken in a fasted state.[138] This makes some people nauseous, however, in which case it should be taken with a meal.

Personally, I train fasted when cutting, and I have 300 milligrams 30 minutes before training and another 300 milligrams a couple of hours before I do cardio later in the day.

YOHIMBINE

Yohimbine is made from the Pausinystalia yohimbe plant, and it helps the body tap into fat stores.[139]

Yohimbine accelerates weight loss, but it only works if you're training in a fasted state. Elevated insulin levels negate yohimbine's effects.[140 141 142]

In terms of dosages, research has shown that 0.2 milligrams per kilogram of body weight is sufficient for fat loss purposes and that ingesting it prior to exercise is particularly effective.[143 144]

Some people get overly jittery from yohimbine, so I recommend that you start with 0.1 milligrams per kilogram of body weight to assess tolerance. If you feel fine, then increase to the clinically effective dosage of 0.2 milligrams per kilogram.

Furthermore, yohimbine can raise blood pressure.[145] If you have high blood pressure, I don't recommend that you use it.

SYNEPHRINE

Synephrine is a chemical compound found in certain types of citrus fruits (particularly the bitter variety).

It's chemically similar to ephedrine and catecholamines (the chemicals adrenaline and noradrenaline, which cause the breakdown of fat cells), and although less potent than those two, it induces similar effects.

Research shows that supplementation with synephrine increases both basal metabolic rate and lipolysis, inhibits the activity of certain types of fat cell receptors that prevent fat mobilization, and increases the thermic effect of food, which is the "energy cost" of metabolizing food.[146 147 148]

Furthermore, research shows that synephrine works synergistically with caffeine to enhance both caffeine's and its own fat loss properties.[149]

Additionally, anything that has the ability to increase catecholamine activity can also suppress hunger between meals (a component of the fight or flight response), and thus synephrine is generally considered to be an appetite suppressant.

Clinically effective dosages of synephrine range from 25 to 50 mg.

Well, that wraps up all the healthy, safe strategies and tricks you can use to make getting shredded as quick and painless as possible.

However, there is one more thing I think we should talk about, and that's how to deal with and control hunger while cutting.

Ideally, you should never get overly hungry while cutting, as this is usually a sign of too severe of a calorie deficit (whether through excessive calorie restriction or exercise, or both). But, for some, a certain degree of hunger at various points in the day is unavoidable and annoying.

Fortunately, there are various ways to effectively reduce hunger, and we'll go over them in the next chapter.

18

EIGHT WAYS TO IMPROVE HUNGER CONTROL AND WEIGHT LOSS

THE #1 WEIGHT-LOSS PROBLEM THAT I help people with is, by far, sticking to their diet.

This is especially the case with people who are new to a healthy weight-loss regimen, which requires that you remain in a caloric deficit for many weeks as opposed to a crash diet that you suffer through for a short period.

The overall experience of being in a caloric deficit varies dramatically. For some (lucky bastards), it causes few or no uncomfortable symptoms: no hunger issues, cravings, or energy lows. For others (the rest of us mere mortals), it can get quite tough due to hunger pangs, intense cravings (usually brought on by simple hunger), and a lingering lethargy (which can be particularly bad when you go low-carb).

What gives? And what can we do to stave off hunger and stick to our diets?

THE SCIENCE OF WEIGHT LOSS AND HUNGER CONTROL

Our natural eating instincts are regulated by three hormones: insulin, ghrelin, and leptin.[150]

When we haven't eaten in several hours and our bodies have finished metabolizing and absorbing the nutrients in our last meal, insulin levels drop to a baseline level (because insulin's job is to shuttle food's nutrients from the blood into the cells for use). Ghrelin levels then rise, which stimulates hunger. When you eat food, leptin levels rise, which turns off the hunger.

Now, when you're in a caloric deficit, circulating leptin levels decrease and ghrelin levels increase.[151] And as you lose body fat, leptin levels drop even further.[152] The net effect of this is dieting for weight loss just generally makes you feel hungrier and makes meals feel less satisfying.

Realize that your body's goal is to attain an energy balance: it wants to match its energy use to its consumption. It doesn't want to be in a deficit. When you listen to your natural instincts and eat more than you planned, it doesn't take much to halt your weight loss. Just a few extra bites of calorie-dense food at each meal can be enough to eliminate the deficit and keep you stuck at your current weight.

That's why keeping hunger under control is so important when dieting for weight loss. If we give in, we fail to lose weight. If we try to suffer through it, we want to run people off the road. Fortunately, defeating hunger isn't too hard when you know what you're doing.

EIGHT SIMPLE, EFFECTIVE DIETARY STRATEGIES TO REDUCE HUNGER

While dieting for weight loss will never be as generally satisfying as eating maintenance calories or a surplus, there are strategies you can use to make it as enjoyable as possible. I use many of these and, knock on wood, find dieting relatively easy and pain-free.

GET 30 TO 40% OF YOUR DAILY ENERGY FROM PROTEIN, AND INCLUDE SOME IN EACH MEAL YOU EAT

When you're dieting to lose weight, protein is your best friend. It helps you preserve muscle and results in basically no fat storage, and research has shown that a high-protein diet reduces overall appetite, possibly by increasing leptin sensitivity (so you feel fuller and more satisfied by the food you eat).[153]

Take advantage of this by getting 30 to 40% of your daily calories from protein, and include some in every meal you eat.

DON'T HEAVILY RESTRICT YOUR CARBOHYDRATE INTAKE

I always hated low-carb dieting because it caused significant declines in strength (due to lower glycogen levels) but also because it just made me generally more hungry. Now I know why.

Dietary fat just isn't very effective at increasing leptin levels, and research has shown that low-carb, high-fat diets reduce 24-hour circulating leptin levels.[154 155] High-fat diets are a recipe for reduced satiety. It's also possible that dietary fat induces leptin resistance (meaning that leptin's signals become blunted), which has been demonstrated in animal research.[156]

Carbohydrates, on the other hand, dramatically increase leptin levels, and the more carbs you eat, the higher your 24-hour circulating leptin levels are.[157 158] A high-protein and moderate-carbohydrate diet makes for a double whammy of satiety.

Based on the above, it's not surprising to find that research has found that high-carbohydrate, low-fat diets are very effective for weight loss, even when subjects ate as much as they wanted each meal.[159] Researchers from the Royal Veterinary and Agricultural University put it simply:

In conclusion, a low-fat diet, high in protein and fibre-rich carbohydrates, mainly from different vegetables, fruits and whole grains, is highly satiating for fewer calories than fatty foods. This diet composition provides good sources of vitamins, minerals, trace elements and fibre, and may have the most beneficial effect on blood lipids and blood-pressure levels.

INCREASE YOUR FIBER INTAKE.

Fiber is an indigestible portion of food that absorbs water as it moves through the digestive tract and helps you take good poops (yup). Research has also shown that it increases satiety.[160]

Keep your fiber intake high by eating plenty of fibrous vegetables and fruits (I include one or the other in every meal). You can even use supplementary fiber like psyllium seed husks, which rapidly expand in your stomach and induce a feeling of fullness.

(And in case you're wondering how much fiber to eat, the Institute of Medicine recommends children and adults consume 14 grams of fiber for every 1,000 calories they eat each day.)[161]

EAT MORE NUTS

Nuts not only contain protein and fiber to increase satiety, but they are a great source of healthy fats as well. Studies have also associated frequent nut consumption with a reduced risk of weight gain.[162]

DRINK WATER WITH EACH MEAL

Research has shown that drinking a couple of glasses of water with each meal increases satiety while eating.[163]

AVOID HIGH-GLYCEMIC CARBOHYDRATES

The glycemic index (or GI) is a scale that measures the effect of different carbohydrates on your blood sugar level.

Carbohydrates that break down slowly and release glucose into the blood slowly are low on the glycemic index. Carbohydrates that break down quickly will release glucose into the blood quickly, causing insulin levels to suddenly spike, and are high on the glycemic index. Below 55 on the GI is considered low and above 70 is considered high. Pure glucose is 100 on the GI.

Research has shown that the rapid absorption of glucose that occurs after eating high-glycemic carbohydrate induces a sequence of hormonal and metabolic changes that result in the desire to eat more.[164]

Furthermore, most high-glycemic foods are processed junk, with little nutritive value. Replace them with unprocessed, low-glycemic alternatives, and you'll be better off in not just the hunger control department but general health as well.

EAT SLOWLY

Research has shown that eating more slowly helps reduce the amount you need to eat to feel satisfied.[165] So take your time, chew your food, and enjoy each bite.

GET ENOUGH SLEEP

When you restrict your sleep, leptin levels drop, and ghrelin levels rise.[166]

One study found that people who slept 5 hours had 15% lower leptin levels and about 15% higher ghrelin levels than people who slept

8 hours.[167] Unsurprisingly, researchers found that the less people slept, the fatter they generally were.

Sleep needs vary from individual to individual, but according to the National Sleep Foundation, adults need 7 to 9 hours of sleep per night to avoid the negative effects of sleep deprivation.

Ultimately, you might not be able to completely banish hunger while dieting, but you should be able to bring it down from downright unbearable to mild and manageable.

And that's how it goes for many people—they use simple tricks to avoid major hunger pangs and learn to deal with the relatively minor feelings of hunger that creep up an hour or so before the next meal.

This chapter wraps up everything that relates to cutting to single-digit body fat percentages. The fun part is next: maintaining a lean physique.

"Fun part?" you might be wondering. Sarcasm?

No—maintenance is quite enjoyable when you do it right.

Contrary to what many "experts" claim and people believe, maintaining low levels of body fat doesn't require that you live on the brink of starvation, avoid all "cheat" foods, or kill yourself in the gym.

If you apply the strategies taught in the next chapter, you'll be able to stay shredded while eating plenty, including the occasional "bad" foods, and spending no more than a handful of hours in the gym each week.

19

HOW TO MAINTAIN SINGLE-DIGIT BODY FAT PERCENTAGES YEAR-ROUND WITH EASE

ONCE YOU'VE PUT IN THE HARD work it takes to get into single-digit body fat percentages, the last thing you want to do is start gaining fat.

Sure, there's the point of vanity—who doesn't like having a six pack?—but your body also feels great when it's lean. You have good energy levels, your body responds well to food you eat, and you enjoy a general sense of well-being that takes the edge off whatever stresses you're facing in life.

That said, what does it take to maintain body fat under 10%?

Do you have to starve yourself or completely write off your social life? (Do you have to be that guy who has already eaten before the party and drinks water all night?)

Can you stay strong while being lean? Can you increase strength and build muscle?

Well, many people believe you have to keep your calories quite low to stay lean and that you simply can't efficiently build muscle or strength with your body fat below 10%.

They're wrong.

If you follow the strategies given in this chapter, you will be able to maintain single-digit body fat percentages for as long as you like while still being able to eat plenty of food, including "cheat" foods.

Furthermore, you'll not only get your pre-cutting strength back, but you'll also be able to make gains and build muscle.

Let's get to it, starting with diet and supplementation.

REVERSE DIETING: THE KEY TO PROPER POST-CUT NUTRITION

What do you want to do once you finish a sub-10% cut? Pound food. Every day. For days and days on end.

I totally understand—I've been there. But it is a big mistake that often leads to rapid fat storage.

Remember that your metabolism is already at a low point at the end of your cut. The worst thing you can do is start bombarding it with thousands of excess calories, as a significant percentage of the overage will be stored as fat.[168] Sure, your metabolism will also speed up, but not enough to offset the influx.

The proper way to go about post-cut dieting is to slowly increase your caloric intake to let your metabolism gradually speed up to a point where you're able to eat a significant amount of food every day without gaining fat.

Just as you have to slowly reduce calories to get shredded, you want to slowly increase them to prevent the dreaded post-cut disappearance of abs, vascularity, and definition that comes with suddenly spiking caloric intake.

Here's how to do it properly:

First, calculate what your TDEE should be given your current weight (remember your actual daily expenditure isn't going to be this high at the end of a cut due to the decrease in your BMR).

To do this, calculate your BMR using the Katch McArdle formula given earlier in the book and multiply it as follows:

- By 1.2 if you exercise 1 to 3 hours per week

- By 1.35 if you exercise 4 to 6 hours per week

- By 1.5 if you exercise 7+ hours per week

This will give you a good approximation of what your TDEE should be at your current weight. This is the number of calories you should be able to eat every day without gaining any fat. (If you're wondering about the difference between training and non-training days, and what to do about it, we'll get to that in a minute.)

You then utilize the reverse dieting protocol given earlier in the book:

Post-Cut Week 1:

Increase your daily calorie intake by 100 by adding 25 grams of carbs to your meal plan.

If you ended your cut at 1,800 calories per day, then you will want to eat 1,900 per day for the next 5 to 7 days.

You want to increase carb intake because our first priority is raising your body's glycogen levels, which are going to be chronically low as a result of the gradual reduction in carbohydrate intake that goes with cutting to the sub-10% range.

Post-Cut Week 2:

Increase your daily calorie intake by 100 by adding 25 grams of carbs to your meal plan.

Same deal as the last. In keeping with the example, your intake would now go up to 2,000 calories per day for 5 to 7 days.

Post-Cut Week 3:

Increase your daily calorie intake by about 100 by adding 10 grams of fat to your meal plan.

Now adjust your fat intake to keep it around 20% of your total daily calories, which ensures hormone production stays in a healthy range, among other things.

Post-Cut Week 4 and Beyond:

Increase your daily calorie intake by 100 by alternating between increasing carbohydrate and fat intake.

You continue this way, increasing daily carbohydrate intake by 25 grams for 5 to 7 days, followed by another carbohydrate intake increase (25 grams more for 5 to 7 days), and followed by the fat intake increase (10 grams more for 5 to 7 days), until you've reached your TDEE for your *current* weight.

This last point is minor but worth addressing. As you do this, your weight will go up. Don't worry, you aren't gaining a bunch of fat; your muscles are simply filling up with glycogen and water.

This can cause more weight gain than some people realize.

My last cut ended around 182 pounds, and over the course of the following 8 weeks, I was able to increase by caloric intake from about 2,000 per day to close to 3,000 per day. During this time, my weight increased to about 192 pounds, with only about a 1 to 1.5% increase in body fat.

You might be wondering why I gained any body fat.

The main reason is I went really hard on some cheat meals. I was honestly just curious how badly I could cheat once or twice per week without gaining noticeable amounts of fat. My highlight was a nearly 5,000-calorie dinner that consisted of a pound of pasta carbonara, 10 ounces of chicken, and two pints (!) of Talenti gelato (nectar of the Gods). I ate around 7,000 calories that day—good times.

Anyway, the bottom line is if I wanted to maintain my absolutely shredded 182-pound look (around 6% body fat), I would have had to stay tighter on my weekly intake, avoiding any large caloric surpluses.

I also find it hard to make steady strength gains when staying this lean. I usually have to undershoot my target TDEE, which means less glycogen in the muscles and less strength.

Therefore, as I don't have any particular reason to stay that lean for extended periods, I generally allow for a bit more weekly calories. Nevertheless, I keep my body fat around 7 to 8%, which is pretty ripped by most standards, and it lets me get back to 5 to 6% within a few weeks of dieting.

MANIPULATING DAILY CALORIC INTAKE TO MAXIMIZE MUSCLE GROWTH WHILE STAYING LEAN

Earlier, when we were talking about calculating TDEE, I mentioned that we would go over the difference between training and rest days.

What I was referring to is simply this: you burn more calories on your training days than rest days, so should you be eating the same number of calories every day (your TDEE), or should training days be higher than rest days?

Fortunately, the answer is simple.

If you take your TDEE number and multiply it by 7, you get your approximate weekly caloric expenditure based on your activity level. So long as you don't grossly overshoot that number in your weekly calorie intake, you won't gain any body fat to speak of.

That said, there are various ways of going about hitting that weekly number.

One is to simply eat the same number of calories every day—your TDEE, as calculated earlier. This is a simple, foolproof way of going about it.

However, I prefer to eat a bit more on my training days and a bit less on my rest days. I have a couple of reasons for doing this:

1. Intense exercise puts increased energy demands on the body, and meeting these demands with adequate intake (at least as many calories as you're burning, preferably a little more) helps maximize muscle growth.[169]

2. The more carbohydrate you eat, the better your performance will be in the gym. Thus, I like my carb intake to be higher on training days than rest days.[170]

Now, I don't just wing it, eating "more" or "less"—I calculate my training and non-training intake targets and stick to them. There are two ways to go about this:

1. Placing yourself in a mild surplus on your training days and a mild deficit on your rest days, balancing them so you match your weekly expenditure.

2. Eating your actual energy expenditure for your training and rest days (true maintenance calories every day).

In my experience, neither is better than the other. It boils down to personal preference and results.

For staying really lean and continuing to make gains in the gym, I prefer #1. But some do better with the second approach. I recommend you try both for 4 to 6 weeks and see which you like best.

Let's now look at how to calculate your daily calories and macronutritient ratios for both methods.

CALCULATING CALORIE INTAKES AND MACRO RATIOS FOR THE SURPLUS/DEFICIT APPROACH

Let's first look at how to set up your diet using my preferred method of the two given above.

1. Start by calculating your weekly intake target. This is simply your TDEE as calculated earlier, multiplied by 7.

2. Your caloric target on your deficit (rest) days is simply your BMR, which will put you in a mild—10 to 15% caloric deficit.

3. Break this daily caloric intake into the following macro ratios: 45% calories from protein, 25% from carbohydrates, and 30% from fats. (One gram of protein and carbohydrate both contain about 4 calories, and one gram of fat contains about 9.) You reduce your carb intake on rest days because you simply don't need the extra carbs, and the increased fat intake is good for increasing insulin sensitivity and boosting anabolic hormone production. [171] [172]

4. Multiply your rest day calories by the number of weekly rest days, and subtract this from your weekly target. This is the total number of calories you will split among your training days.

5. Divide the sum by the number of weekly training days for your caloric target on your training days.

6. Break this daily caloric intake into the following macro ratios: 1 gram of protein per pound of body weight, 20% of calories from fats, and the rest from carbohydrate.

7. Work your meal plan over so you hit these daily targets. To make this easier, I like to stick to the same types of foods but increase or decrease portions to fit my intake needs.

This might sound complicated, but it's actually quite simple. Here's an example (I round numbers up/down to keep things simple, making sure I'm not rounding all up):

	Me	**You**
Weekly Calorie Expenditure		
(Intake Target) .... 2,800 x 7 = 19,600		_____
Training Days...5		_____
Rest Days 2		_____
Rest Day Calories (BMR) .... 2,100 calories		_____
Rest Day Macros (2,100 x 0.45) / 4 = 240 g protein		_____
(2,100 x 0.25) / 4 = 130 g carbs		_____
(2,100 x 0.30) / 9 = 70 g fat		_____
My Weekly Rest Day Calories...................................4200		_____
Weekly Training Day Calories 19,600 – 4,200 = 15,400		_____
Training Day Calories......................... 15,400 / 5 = 3,100		_____
Training Day Macros My Body Weight = 190 g protein		_____
(3,100 x 0.20) / 9 = 70 g fat		_____
(3,100 - ((190 x 4) + (70 x 9)) / 4 = 430 g carbs		_____

(In case you're wondering how I calculated the carbs, I simply subtracted my protein and fat calories from the daily total, and divided that by 4.)

So, all I have to do is eat 190 grams protein, 430 grams carbs, and 70 grams fat on my training days, and 240 grams protein, 130 grams carbs, and 70 grams fat on my rest days, and I will be able to not only stay lean but also continue to build muscle and strength.

A training day, by the way, is a day on which you lift. If you only do cardio, treat this as a rest day (a little larger deficit won't hurt).

The above formula works well so long as you're lifting at least 3 days per week. If you're only lifting 1 or 2 days per week, then you modify it as follows:

1. Eat TDEE + 20% on lifting days using the same macro breakdown given above: 1 gram of protein per pound of body weight, 20% of calories from fat, and the rest from carbohydrate.

2. Split the remaining weekly calories evenly across the remaining days: 1 gram of protein per pound of body weight, 30% of daily calories from fat, and the rest from carbohydrate.

So, for example:

My Weekly Calorie Expenditure
(Intake Target) ....2,800 * 7 = 19,600
My Training Days 2
My Training Day Calories.. 3,400
My Weekly Training Day Calories.............................. 6,800
My Weekly Remaining Calories 12,800
My No-Training Day Calories..................................... 2,600

Simple enough. (I skipped the macro calculations because I don't think you need to run through them again.)

Calculating Calorie Intakes and Macro Ratios for the True TDEE Approach

Let's now look at how to work out your diet using the second of the two approaches where you eat (more or less) the same amount of calories as you burn each day. You probably already know how to calculate this, but let's run through it quickly.

1. Start by calculating your weekly intake target as calculated earlier.

2. Your caloric target on your rest days is your BMR multiplied by 1.1, which will put you right around maintenance calories for the day.

3. Break this daily caloric intake into the following macro ratios: 45% calories from protein, 25% from carbohydrates, and 30% from fats.

    Again, we are reducing your carb intake for reasons given earlier.

4. Multiply your rest day calories by the number of weekly rest days, and subtract this from your weekly target. This is the total number of calories you will split among your training days.

5. Divide the sum by the number of weekly training days for your daily caloric target for your training days.

6. Break this daily caloric intake into the following macro ratios: 1 gram of protein per pound of body weight, 20% of calories from fat, and the rest from carbohydrate.

7. Work your meal plan over so you hit these daily targets.

Again, an example:

My Weekly Calorie Expenditure
(Intake Target) ....2,800 x 7 = 19,600
My Training Days 5
My Rest Days...2
My Rest Day Calories
(BMR * 1.1) .... 2,300 calories
My Weekly Rest Day Calories..4,600
My Weekly Training Day
Calories..19,600 – 4,600 = 15,000
My Training Day
Calories.. 15,000 / 5 = 3,000

Again, I'll skip the macro calculations, but that's all there is to it.

HOW TO EAT WHEN YOU'RE NOT TRAINING

If you're taking a Rest Week or are unable to get into the gym for whatever reason, I recommend you keep your calories at a maintenance level and reduce your carbohydrate intake.

For your calories, calculate them by multiplying your BMR by 1.1 (or 1.15 if you're moving around a fair amount every day).

For your macros, get 40% of your calories from protein, 30% from carbohydrates, and 30% from fats.

Simple enough.

HOW TO EAT ON A DELOAD WEEK

When you deload, do the following:

• On the days you don't train, use the above formula for intake.

• On the days you do train, calculate your intake by multiplying your BMR by 1.25 and get 40% of calories from protein, 40%

from carbohydrates, and 20% from fats.

HOW TO CHEAT WITHOUT GETTING FAT

So, you now know the secret to manipulating your daily caloric intakes to allow for unimpaired muscle and strength gains without adding body fat.

What about cheating, though?

That is, what about having a social life? Going out to dinner with your girlfriend or wife? Enjoying yourself at a birthday party? Is it all hopeless? Do you have to be that guy who has always already eaten, turning away drinks and goodies?

Nope, you don't.

Here is the simplest way to deal with such situations:

You save up calories/macros for the upcoming feast by eating nothing but protein leading up to it. Skip post-workout carbs and everything else—just have protein all day. You eat protein on your normal feeding schedule or follow an intermittent fasting routine for the day, fasting up until about 8 hours before the feast.

If this is a training day, you can easily come into such an occasion with a huge amount of food you have to eat just to hit your daily numbers. (If you can eat 250+ grams of carbs and 80+ grams of fat in one meal and still want more, you're a beast.)

When I do this, I don't go OCD on tracking every little thing I eat—I just keep a good estimated running count in my head and cut it off somewhere around my numbers.

And if you go off the deep end and binge, don't sweat it. Chances are you won't even notice a difference. If you're particularly paranoid, you can simply go into a deficit on 2 or 3 of your training days by eating 20% fewer calories on those days than you normally would have.

Another little trick for cheating while staying really lean is to burn up some glycogen before the feast. You best accomplish this by weightlifting or by performing HIIT cardio (shoot for 20 to 30 minutes).[173]

When your body is in this glycogen-depleted state, its ability to replenish glycogen stores is greatly increased.[174] In this state, your muscles can supercompensate with glycogen, meaning they can store more than they had before the depletion.

This creates a nice "carb sink" that you can fill without having to worry about fat storage, because the body will not store carbohydrate as fat until glycogen stores are replenished.[175]

SUPPLEMENTATION AND STAYING SUPER LEAN

Fortunately, supplements don't play a big role in staying really lean.

I don't take fat burners, caffeine pills, or yohimbine when maintaining, but I do take green tea extract for its weight maintenance effects and its other health benefits (as discussed in *BLS*).

However, I do take a couple of supplements that, among other things, help maintain optimal insulin sensitivity.

THE ROLE OF INSULIN SENSITIVITY IN STAYING LEAN AND BUILDING MUSCLE

As you know, insulin sensitivity refers to how well your cells respond to insulin's signals to accept nutrients from food you've eaten.

Insulin resistance, on the other hand, is just that: the cells failing to respond to insulin's signals. And this impairs your body's ability to burn fat, increases the likelihood that it will store carbohydrates as fat and suppresses intracellular signaling responsible for protein synthesis.[176 177]

In simple terms, the more insulin resistant your body is, the easier it is to get fatter, and the harder it is to build muscle. On other hand, the better your body's insulin sensitivity, the easier it is to stay lean and build muscle.

Thus, keeping insulin sensitivity as high as possible is a big help when you want to stay really lean. Fortunately, regular exercise and simply being lean does wonders for insulin sensitivity, but there's more you can do.

On the dietary side, you can reduce carbohydrate intake a couple of days per week, as we discussed earlier.

However, I don't recommend following a low-carb diet on your training days for a few reasons:

- Carbohydrates supply our body with the molecules needed to synthesize glycogen, which improves physical performance.[178 179]

Building muscle strength and size requires that we continually push our muscles harder and harder (progressive overload), and this is essentially impossible when our glycogen levels are chronically low (which is one of the byproducts of reducing carbohydrate intake).

- Research has shown that when muscle glycogen levels are low, exercise-induced muscle breakdown is accelerated.[180] Why is that bad? Aren't we trying to break down our muscles with exercise?

Yes, but remember that our body can only synthesize so many muscle proteins every day. If we cause too much damage with our exercise, our body simply won't be able to keep up with repair, which can result in us losing muscle despite regular training.

- Carbohydrates stimulate the production of insulin, which doesn't induce protein synthesis but does inhibit protein breakdown and thus affects overall muscle growth. One study compared high- vs. low-carbohydrate dieting and found that subjects following the low-carb diet had increased protein degradation and reduced protein synthesis rates, resulting is less overall muscle growth.[181] [182]

The bottom line is while low-carb dieting has benefits for those with impaired glucose metabolism (diabetics or pre-diabetics, for example), it is not good for maximizing muscle growth.[183]

Intermittent fasting (IF) is also a good way to improve insulin sensitivity.[184] If you're not familiar with this dietary protocol, we'll be covering it in depth in a later chapter.

I like to use IF on my rest days. To do this, I simply eat my last meal around 8 PM the night before and don't eat again until 12 PM the next day.

I also use stevia to sweeten the tea I like to drink every day, and I include cinnamon in my post-workout shake, both of which have been shown to improve insulin sensitivity.[185] [186]

On the supplementation side, green tea extract has been shown to increase insulin sensitivity in animal research,[187] fish oil is well known for its effectiveness in this regard,[188] and spirulina can have this effect as well.[189] I supplement with these every day, as they also confer many other health benefits.

TRAINING TIPS FOR MAINTAINING SINGLE-PERCENT BODY FAT PERCENTAGES

I saved this for last because, well, there isn't much to say.

Staying really lean is primarily a matter of properly controlling your diet. You don't have to do anything special in terms of training beyond adjusting your caloric intake to your training frequency.

My normal maintenance training schedule is lifting 5 or 6 times per week for about 45 to 60 minutes each session and doing cardio 3 times per week for about 25 minutes per session.

Cardio isn't necessary for staying really lean, but it's good for the body, and being able to eat more food throughout the week is nice. I prefer HIIT cardio, but sometimes will do LISS if my legs are too sore from my lifting.

In your lifting, go heavy and hard with the intention of making progress, not just maintaining strength. You should have no trouble building both strength and muscle, albeit slowly, while staying lean.

Well, that wraps up the subject of staying shredded with ease.

In the next few chapters, we're going to talk about a few different dietary protocols that you've probably heard of and that you may be interested in knowing more about. We'll go over how they work and when and why you may want to use them.

We're going to start with intermittent fasting, as it's particularly popular these days.

20

THE DEFINITIVE GUIDE TO
INTERMITTENT FASTING

GENERALLY SPEAKING, THE BEST WAY TO avoid the scams and pitfalls of the health and fitness industry is to simply ignore the latest and greatest methods of losing weight or building muscle.

Eat healthfully and regulate your calories, engage in regular resistance and cardiovascular exercise, and save your money on the junk peddled by Dr. Oz, and you will do just fine.

Every so often, true advances in this industry do occur, though.

- It was long believed that eating saturated fats increased your risk of heart disease. We now know that's not true. [190]

- It was once thought that high-protein diets wreck your kidneys. Well, they don't, and they actually are quite healthy. [191][192]

- Even the still-trendy dogma that eating carbohydrates will automatically make you fat is on its way out.

As scientists learn more and more about how the human body works and how to manipulate it, genuine breakthroughs are made that help us improve our physiques and live longer, healthier lives.

Is intermittent fasting one of these breakthroughs? Or is it just another way to sell magazines, books, and workout products? Let's find out.

THE BASICS OF INTERMITTENT FASTING

Intermittent fasting (or IF as many people call it) is a style of dieting that revolves around restricting your eating for extended periods of time and then eating your day's worth of food during predetermined feeding windows.

For instance, you might fast (eat nothing) for 16 hours per day and eat during the remaining 8 hours. Or you might fast for 20 hours per day and cram all your calories into a 4-hour window. Some protocols even call for eating one day and fasting the next.

Why bother with such a diet? According to some, it's the way of the future. They say it makes losing fat and building muscle easier than ever and that it'll help you live longer, ward off disease, skyrocket your anabolic hormones, and accelerate your metabolism to incredible speeds—all while eating large meals and, according to some of the sleazier "gurus," eating basically whatever you want.

Well, when things sound too good to be true, they almost always are.

Intermittent fasting won't turn you into a superhuman, but fasting itself has plenty of health benefits. So let's dive in, starting with the perceived evils of fasting.

FASTING AND MUSCLE LOSS

If this style of dieting sounds like a recipe for muscle disaster to you, I understand.

Like everyone, I once believed that going longer than 4 or 5 hours without food—and protein in particular—would result in muscle loss and metabolic slowdown. I stuck to my protein intake schedule religiously and would get "hangry" (hungry + angry) if I had to go for more than 4 hours without eating anything.

Well, this is a myth that the rising popularity of intermittent fasting has completely blown out of the water. Some people just throw out a study showing that intermittent fasting doesn't affect whole-body protein metabolism any differently than traditional forms of dieting and declare themselves the victor, but I want to go deeper than that.[193]

I want to explain why this is, because I think it will help you in your dieting, regardless of whether you give intermittent fasting a go.

So, let's start with why your body would even break muscle down in the first place.

Glucose, or blood sugar, is a great source of energy for your cells and organs. Your brain particularly likes glucose and is quite a hog—research has shown that it uses more than 25% of total body glucose.[194]

The easiest way to provide your body with glucose is to eat carbohydrate, but your body is also able to create it out of other substances, such as amino acids and glycerol (found in body fat) via a process known as gluconeogenesis.

When you're in a fasted state—when your body is no longer absorbing nutrients from your last meal and is now relying on its energy stores—your body has two primary sources of glucose:

1. Glycogen stores in the liver, which are broken down into glucose and released into the blood for use

2. Body fat, which is broken down into free fatty acids that can be used as energy by many of your cells, and glycerol, which can be converted into glucose

These two sources keep everything working as usual, with absolutely no cannibalizing of muscle.

Now, the liver runs out of glycogen after anywhere from 6 to 24 hours of fasting (the time to exhaustion varies based on your body's glucose needs, basal metabolic rate, and more). As the liver's stores deplete, the body will begin to look for amino acids to convert into glucose. If none are available in the blood, it will break down muscle to get them.

Unfortunately, there's a distinct lack of good research in this field, but the work of Dr. George F. Cahill lends insight. He found that amino acids from muscle were responsible for about 50% of glucose maintenance at the 16-hour mark of fasting and 100% at the 28-hour mark.[195]

The bottom line is the body wants to spare muscle whenever possible, and in most cases, no serious muscle loss can occur until you've fasted for 12 to 16 hours. (I'd also like to note that physical activity would cause this to happen faster, of course, because it would put greater energy demands on the body.)

BUT WAIT…there's more.

I'd like to repeat something and comment on it: the body will use amino acids in the blood for *gluconeogenesis* over *breaking down its own muscle.*

Why is that important?

Because when you eat protein, it can result in a steady release of amino acids for many, many hours.[196] So if you eat a meal full of slow-burning proteins, such as casein or egg, and you then fast for 12 to 16 hours, your body is going to have plenty of free amino acids available in the blood for conversion into glucose. Cannibalizing muscle won't be necessary.

FASTING AND STARVATION MODE

We've all heard about starvation mode, and it seems to make logical sense at first.

If we go too long without eating, wouldn't our body think it's being starved and drastically reduce its metabolic speed? To better deal with future starvations, wouldn't it increase the rate at which it stores fat once we do eat?

Well, regardless of how much it might seem theoretically plausible, it's not true.

A study conducted by researchers at the University of Rochester showed that metabolic rate didn't decline until *60 hours* of fasting…and the reduction was a mere 8%.[197] In fact, research has demonstrated that the metabolism speeds up after 36 to 48 hours of fasting.[198]

If we look at it, this makes sense from an evolutionary perspective. If we haven't eaten in quite some time, what does our body want us to do? Go find food, of course. And how does it stimulate us to do that?

By increasing production of two chemicals called adrenaline and noradrenaline, which sharpen our minds and make us want to go move around. They also increase our BMR (exercise elevates these chemicals as well).

True starvation in the eyes of the body occurs at about 3 days (72 hours) of not eating, at which point the primary source of energy becomes the breakdown of proteins (and the biggest source of protein is muscle).[199]

Once this occurs, the body knows its survival is imperiled, because what happens when we lose muscle? We become physically weaker, our metabolism slows down, we become more likely to succumb to disease, and, eventually, we die (and usually from heart attack).

So, don't worry—incorporating some fasting into your meal scheduling won't wreck your metabolism.

THE BENEFITS OF FASTING

Now that we have the big bad myths of fasting behind us, let's talk about some of its benefits.

- Research conducted by scientists at the University of California demonstrated that alternate-day fasting decreased blood pressure, reduced oxidative damage to various tissues and DNA, improved insulin sensitivity and glucose uptake, and decreased fat mass.[200]

- A study conducted by researchers at the University Hospital of South Manchester demonstrated that weight loss using an intermittent fasting protocol resulted in greater improvements in insulin sensitivity than a traditional, continuous energy diet.[201]

- Researchers at the University of Virginia found that fasting elevates growth hormone levels (up to five-fold at the 40-hour mark of fasting).[202]

- According to research conducted by the University of Leuven, exercising in a fasted state accelerates fat loss.[203]

- Animal research conducted by the Gerontology Research Center found that increasing time between meals can improve brain health.[204]

- A study conducted by researchers at the Maltepe University School of Medicine found that intermittent fasting reduced inflammation biomarkers.[205]

- Fasting induces autophagy, which is the process whereby your cells eliminate waste material and repair themselves. Autophagy is a crucial part of maintaining muscle mass and fighting the degenerative aspects of aging.[206] [207] (In fact, autophagy is the primary anti-aging mechanism of calorie restriction, which has made headlines these days for its anti-aging benefits.)

The bottom line is fasting is good for the body. It's like a systemic reset button, allowing for the disposal of waste and the reparation of cells and the optimization of the body's many processes.

SHOULD WE ALL BE FOLLOWING AN INTERMITTENT FASTING DIET, THEN?

At this point, you're probably expecting me to say that intermittent fasting truly is the way to go. Well, there's more to the story.

Intermittent fasting is still in its scientific infancy, with only a handful of controlled human studies under its belt.

Sure, we know that fasting itself has health benefits, and we know that intermittent fasting protocols work in terms of losing fat and building muscle, but the real question is, Do they work better than traditional, continuous energy diets?

And that's where we just don't have enough research to know.

For instance, intermittent fasting proponents will often tout a study conducted by the USDA as conclusive proof that they have a better mousetrap.[208] This study showed that men eating one meal per day lost more weight than those who ate three and gained some muscle to boot. Game, set, match, punk.[209]

Well, hold on a minute.

If you read the entire study, you'll quickly see it has some serious flaws:

- A small sample size (15 participants completed the trial)

- A short duration (2-week lead-in and 6-week treatment period)

- A 28% dropout rate (Why did so many people quit?)

- And the worst, the use of bioelectrical impedance analysis (BIA) for body composition (which is notoriously inaccurate—one study using BIA showed that 42 days of fasting caused a 32% decrease in body fat and gains in lean mass…yeah, okay)[210]

Considering the above, the results of the USDA study are essentially worthless.

Another very important point you must realize is that exercising alone provides many of the health benefits associated with intermittent fasting.[211] If you're obese, hate moving, and want to lose weight and get healthier, then intermittent fasting is probably a good way to go. If you're a healthy adult who exercises regularly, however, will it provide any benefits over a traditional meal pattern? *Nobody knows yet.*

On an anecdotal note, I've both tried intermittent fasting routines and worked with many people who have, and I've yet to see anything notably different in terms of results. Yes, it works—you can use it to build muscle or lose fat. But no, I don't believe it's the Holy Grail of dieting that allows you to get bigger and leaner regardless of how long you've been training and your current conditioning. Only newbie gains and steroids can do that.

Another common issue is hunger control, especially when in a caloric deficit. Some people get *really* hungry after 10 to 12 hours of fasting and find it very hard to go any longer. I don't see any good reason for them to continue trying to jam the square peg into the round hole—they should just increase meal frequency until they find a nice sweet spot for their bodies.

If you're a healthy adult who exercises regularly, whether you should follow an intermittent fasting protocol just boils down to how you like to eat and what best fits your lifestyle.

I hate the excessive fullness and lethargy that follows a large meal, and my schedule doesn't lend itself well to shorter feeding windows. Thus, intermittent fasting isn't for me.

However, I know people who don't mind eating large meals and who find reducing meal frequency helps them stick to their diets. Intermittent fasting works well for them.

Even if you enjoy a more traditional style of dieting like I do, you can work in a planned fast once or twice per week. I occasionally do by simply skipping breakfast on a day that I'm not lifting (I lift early in the morning) and eating my first meal after about 12 to 14 hours of fasting. Whether doing this once or twice per week has any real health benefits is up in the air, but I do enjoy how it feels, so that counts for something.

THE POPULAR
INTERMITTENT FASTING PROTOCOLS

Let's now review some of the more popular intermittent fasting methods out there and who they work best for.

LEANGAINS

This method was created and popularized by Martin Berkhan, and it works like this:

- You fast for 16 hours per day. That means no food, but coffee, tea, and non-caloric beverages are fine.

- You have an 8-hour daily feeding window.

- You eat a lot of protein.

- You eat more carbs and calories on training days and more fat and fewer calories on rest days.

- Your post-workout meal is absolutely huge—about 50% of your daily calories.

The Leangains method was built specifically for weightlifters and for people who care about their body composition. If that's you, then I recommend you use it over the other options I discuss here.

It has a few more moving parts than what I've outlined above, so I'll just share Mr. Berkhan's own explanation from his website:[212]

FASTING AND FEEDING

"My general position on the fasted phase is that it should last through the night and during the morning hours. Ideally the fast should then be broken at noon or shortly thereafter if you arise at 6-7 AM like most people. Afternoons and evenings are usually spent in the fed state.

"However, the fast could also also be broken later in the day depending on your personal preferences and daily routine. I personally tend to break the fast as late as 4-6 PM since I work well into the night and rise later than most people with normal jobs.

"The recommendation for fasting through the earlier part of the day, as opposed to the latter part of the day, is for behavioral and social reasons. Most people simply find it easier to fast after awakening and prefer going to bed satiated. Afternoons and evenings are times to unwind and eat. For adherence reasons during dieting, I've also found that placing the feeding phase later in the day is ideal for most people.

THE PROTOCOLS

"I work with four different protocols depending on when my clients train. Depending on setup, one, two, or three meals are eaten in the post-workout period.

FASTED TRAINING

"Training is initiated on an empty stomach and after ingestion of 10 g BCAA or similar amino acid mixture. This "pre-workout" meal is not counted towards the feeding phase. Technically, training is not completely fasted - that would be detrimental. The pre-workout protein intake, with its stimulatory effect on protein synthesis and metabolism, is a crucial compromise to optimize results. The 8-hour feeding phase starts with the post-workout meal.

"*Sample setup*

"*11:30-12 AM or 5-15 minutes pre-workout: 10 g BCAA*

"*12-1 PM: Training*

"*1 PM: Post-workout meal (largest meal of the day)*

"*4 PM: Second meal*

"*9 PM: Last meal before the fast*

"Calories and carbs are tapered down throughout the day in the example above.

EARLY MORNING FASTED TRAINING

"Here's a sample setup for a client that trains early in the morning and prefers the feeding phase at noon or later:

"6 AM: 5-15 minutes pre-workout: 10 g BCAA

"6-7 AM: Training

"8 AM: 10 g BCAA

"10 AM: 10 g BCAA

"12-1 PM: The "real" post-workout meal (largest meal of the day). Start of the 8 hour feeding-window

"8-9 PM: Last meal before the fast

"For the sake of convenience, I recommend getting BCAA in the form of powder and not tabs. Simply mix 30 g of BCAA powder in a shake and drink one third of it every other hour starting 5-15 minutes pre-workout. Tabs are cheaper, but much more of a hassle (you're going to have to pop a lot of tabs).

ONE PRE-WORKOUT MEAL

"This is the most common setup for my younger clients that are still in college or have flexible working hours.

"Sample setup

"12-1 PM or around lunch/noon: Pre-workout meal. Approximately 20-25% of daily total calorie intake

"3-4 PM: Training should happen a few hours after the pre-workout meal.

"4-5 PM: Post-workout meal (largest meal)

"8-9 PM: Last meal before the fast

TWO PRE-WORKOUT MEALS

"This is the usual protocol for people with normal working hours:

"Sample setup

"12-1 PM or around lunch/noon: Meal one. Approximately 20-25% of daily total calorie intake

"4-5 PM: Pre-workout meal. Roughly equal to the first meal
"8-9 PM: Post-workout meal (largest meal)

"Key Points :

- "No calories are to be ingested during the fasted phase, though coffee, calorie free sweeteners, diet soda and sugar free gum are ok (even though they might contain trace amount of calories). A tiny splash of milk in your coffee won't affect anything either (½-1 teaspoon of milk per cup at the most - use sparingly and sensibly if you drink a lot of coffee). Neither will sugar free gum in moderation (~20 g).

- "The fast is the perfect time to be productive and get things done. Don't sit around, get bored and brood about food.

- "Meal frequency during the feeding phase is irrelevant. However, most people, including me, prefer three meals.

- "The majority of your daily calorie intake is consumed in the post-workout period. Depending on setup, this means that approximately 95-99% (fasted training), 80% (one pre-workout meal) or 60% (two pre-workout meals) of your daily calorie intake is consumed after training.

- "The feeding window should be kept somewhat constant due to the hormonal entrainment of meal patterns. We tend to get hungry when we're used to eating and maintaining a regular pattern makes diet adherence easier. If you're used to breaking the fast at 12-2 PM and ending it at 8-10 PM, then try to maintain that pattern every day.

- "On rest days, meal one should ideally be the largest meal, as opposed to training days where the post-workout meal is the largest meal. A good rule of thumb is to make meal one on rest days at least 35-40% of your daily calorie intake. This meal should be very high in protein; some of my clients consume more than 100 g of protein in this meal.

- "When working with clients I am always open to compromising on the above rule. If your preference is to eat a larger meal in the evening instead of noon, or whenever you break the fast, it's no great harm. Some people prefer to save the largest meal on rest days for dinner with their family instead of having a large lunch and that's fine by me if it makes them enjoy and adhere to their diet better.

- "Macronutrients and calorie intakes are always cycled through the week. The specifics depends on the client's ultimate goal: fat loss, muscle gain or body recomposition. Generally speaking, carbs and total calorie intake is highest on training days. On rest days, carbs are lower and fat is higher. Protein is kept high on all days.

- "Here are the supplements I recommend everyone to take on a daily basis: a multivitamin, fish oil, vitamin D and extra calcium (unless dairy is consumed on a regular and daily basis).

- "For fasted training, BCAA or an essential amino acid mixture is highly recommended. However, if this feels like too much micromanaging or simply questionable from an economic standpoint, you could also make due with some whey protein.

- "People sometimes ask me which protocol is best. I tend to look at things from a behavioral perspective first and foremost, so my reply to that is to choose the protocol best suited to your daily routine and training preferences. When dealing with clients I make the choice for them. If you work a 9-5 job and your only option is to train after work, training fasted is generally a bad idea and I always choose the one or two meals pre-workout protocol.

- "Even from a physiological perspective, each protocol has it's own strengths and theoretical benefits. With "physiological perspective" I mean in terms of nutrient partition-

> ing, fat loss and muscle growth. This deserves an article on it's own. I have some interesting and compelling arguments that I think are very unique."

EAT STOP EAT

This method was put together by Brad Pilon, and it's very simple:

- Once or twice per week, fast for 24 hours. Start it whenever you want in the day, but you have to go for 24 hours without eating.

- Break your fast with a normal meal. Don't try to make up for the calories you would've normally eaten the day before.

- Exercise regularly.

This method is better suited to people who want to reap some of the health benefits of fasting but aren't too concerned with body composition (aren't regular, dedicated weightlifters). Be warned, however: going 24 hours without food can be tough, even for people who generally do well with fasting.

THE WARRIOR DIET

This is Ori Hofmekler's method, popularized by his book:

- Eat one massive meal per day, ideally at night. You have 3 to 4 hours to eat, so you're looking at a 20-hour fast followed by a 4-hour feeding window.

- You can have a little bit of fruit and veggies during the day, but little to no protein until your night feast.

- Exercise should be done during the day, in a fasted state.

People who have trouble going for longer periods without food will find this easier because of the light snacking leading up to the feast, but this technically isn't fasting, so this method seems wonky.

ALTERNATE-DAY FASTING

This is similar to Eat Stop Eat. It goes like this:

- Eat normally one day, having your last meal at night.

- Don't eat the next day.

- Start eating the following day at the time you had your last meal.

So if you ate your last meal at 9 PM on Monday, you then fast Tuesday and resume eating at 9 AM Wednesday. Yes, that's a 36-hour fast.

I would only recommend this to people with health problems who are interested in the therapeutic benefits of prolonged fasting periods (20+ hours).

This style of dieting requires that you go to bed on an empty stomach after 24 hours of fasting, which will be particularly rough for most. As you know, there are also muscle loss issues that come into play when you fast for this long.

EAT WHEN YOU'RE HUNGRY, OR WHEN YOU CAN

The simplest way to incorporate fasting into your diet is to simply eat when you feel like it or when you can.

For instance, if you wake up and you're not hungry, don't think you have to eat just for the sake of eating. Fast for a few hours and then have a meal when you're hungry. If you find yourself stuck in a situation where the only food available is fast food and other greasy junk, skip the meal and make it up later.

Knowing that you can fast and eat when you feel like it can be useful because it gives you flexibility in hitting your daily macronutritional targets. For instance, if I skipped my morning meals that would've consisted of about 50 grams of protein, 60 grams of carbs, and 20 grams of fat, that's fairly easy to work into my other meals so I can ensure I don't undereat.

ADDITIONAL THOUGHTS AND OBSERVATIONS ON INTERMITTENT FASTING

So long as you hit proper macronutritional numbers every day, intermittent fasting works. You can use it to lose fat or build muscle.

That said, there are a few potential downsides that you should know about:

- Some people have a lot of trouble fasting and wind up anxious and hungry as they come into the final hour or two before they can eat. Furthermore, women seem to have a harder time fasting than men. They get much hungrier much quicker despite using the hunger control strategies given earlier in the book. In the end, this style of dieting just isn't for everyone.

- Some people, like me, don't like having to eat fewer, larger meals. I don't like the post-meal lethargy that comes with having to eat 700 to 1,000 calories in one go; I much prefer eating 5 to 7 smaller meals each day, with a variety of foods.

- Regardless of your meal size preferences, due to the amount of food you're eating every day, it is pretty uncomfortable for most when they're bulking. If you're cutting, you don't have to fit too many calories into your eating window, and thus your meals are manageable. When you're bulking, it becomes a challenge. Your meals are really big, and your post-workout meal in particular is a behemoth (as you're eating 30 to 40% of your daily calories in this meal).

The bottom line is if the idea of eating fewer, larger meals every day sounds appealing, then you may want to give intermittent fasting a try. If not, then it's probably not going to be for you.

Another circumstance in which I would recommend you give intermittent fasting a try is if, despite using all the strategies discussed in the chapter on getting really lean, you still are having trouble getting there. Intermittent fasting can be particularly good for helping get rid of the last bits of stubborn fat.

Now, let's move on to the next dietary protocol I'd like to cover, which is known as carb cycling.

Like intermittent fasting, carb cycling is quite popular in bodybuilding circles, but it is also quite misunderstood by many gym-goers. It's not the secret to rapid weight loss like some claim, but it does have its uses.

21

THE DEFINITIVE GUIDE
TO CARB CYCLING

LIKE INTERMITTENT FASTING, THE CARB-CYCLING diet has some pretty big shoes to fill if you listen to its more fervent advocates.

According to them, carb cycling delivers the Holy Grail of bodybuilding: rapid fat loss while preserving, or even building, muscle.

The more ridiculous claims go even further, enticing you with promises that you won't have to count calories and the allure of the high-carb day, wherein you stuff yourself silly with precious carbohydrates.

Another common selling point of the carb-cycling diet is the claim that a traditional approach to dieting (steady protein, carbohydrate, and fat intake throughout the week, with planned cheats/refeeds) simply can't get you to the super-lean category (7% and under for men, 16% and under for women) without burning up a ton of muscle.

Well, in this chapter, we'll not only dive into what carb cycling is and how you do it, but we'll also cut through the hype and hyperbole surrounding the matter and use science and anecdotal experience to get at its heart.

WHAT IS THE CARB-CYCLING DIET?

The carb-cycling diet is very simple. It works like this:

- Throughout the week, you rotate through high-carb, moderate-carb, and low/no-carb days.

- All days require a high protein intake.

- Your fat intake is inversely related to your carbohydrate intake. That is, your fat intake is low when your carbs are high, and vice versa.

Exact protocols vary in terms of specific numbers, but all are based on that simple structure.

For example, you may do 4 low-carb days, followed by a high-carb day, and then a no-carb day, and then start over. Or you may do 3 low-carb days followed by 1 high-carb day, and then back to the low-carb and so on.

Here's what these days often look like numerically:

- A high-carb day will generally have you eating 2 to 2.5 grams of carbohydrate per pound of body weight. Your protein intake will be around 1 gram per pound, and your fat intake will be as low as possible (just the fats that come along with lean proteins, but no high-fat foods like oils, nuts, butter, eggs, and so forth).

- A moderate-carb day will call for about 1.5 grams of carbohydrate per pound of body weight. Your protein intake will be between 1 and 1.2 grams per pound, and your fat intake will be around 0.2 grams per pound.

- A low-carb day will call for about 0.5 grams of carbohydrate per pound of body weight. Your protein intake will usually increase to about 1.5 grams per pound, and your fat intake will increase to around 0.35 grams per pound.

- A no-carb day means fewer than 30 grams of carbohydrate. To achieve this, you basically can only eat a few servings of vegetables per day. Protein intake is around 1.5 grams per pound, and fat intake goes up to 0.5 to 0.8 grams per pound.

The theory behind the diet is as follows:

Your high-carb day will refuel your muscles' glycogen levels and flood your body with insulin, which has anti-catabolic effects (but not true anabolic effects like some people claim—insulin does not induce protein synthesis and instead inhibits muscle breakdown).[213][214] Most protocols recommend that you do your toughest workout on your high-carb day.

Your moderate-carb day gives you plenty of carbs to maintain glycogen stores, but it doesn't put you in enough of a caloric deficit to cause much weight loss. You train on these days.

Your no- and low-carb days are the days where you're in a caloric deficit and where some people claim the magic happens. These are the days where you trick your body into burning fat at an accelerated rate by keeping insulin levels low.

It's usually recommended that you use cardio or rest days for no/low-carb days, but if you lift more than 3 days per week, you will have to lift on 1 or more of these days (which sucks).

So, that's how to do it. Let's address the next question on your mind: Does it work?

IS CARB CYCLING GOOD FOR WEIGHT LOSS?

Can you use carb cycling to lose fat? Absolutely.

Any dietary protocol that puts you in a calorie deficit, whether it's daily or weekly or even monthly, will result in weight loss, regardless of the macronutrient breakdown.[215]

Part of the appeal of carb cycling is the claim that you don't have to count calories or watch what you eat. You simply follow a set of simple rules regarding eating a lot of carbs on high days, fewer on moderate days, and very few on no/low days.

This loose style of dieting works decently for maintenance and may work for weight loss to a degree, but it never works for getting shredded.

Getting below 8 or 9% body fat (men) or 18 or 19% (women) requires that you plan and track your macronutrient intake closely. Period.

You need to know exactly how much protein, carbohydrate, and fat you're eating every day, and you need to manipulate these numbers to keep yourself in enough of a calorie deficit to continue losing fat, but not so much that you sacrifice muscle.

So the question of carb cycling and weight loss becomes…

IS CARB CYCLING BETTER FOR WEIGHT LOSS THAN TRADITIONAL DIETING?

Enthusiasts of the carb-cycling diet will claim that your low-carb days will greatly accelerate your fat loss over what it would be with a traditional approach to dieting.

Unfortunately, science isn't on their side. As you know, reducing carbohydrate intake doesn't always accelerate fat loss—it depends how your body deals with carbohydrates.

Particularly relevant to this chapter is another study conducted by researchers at Arizona State University, wherein researchers pitted a ketogenic diet (a very low-carbohydrate diet) versus a traditional diet to see whether one had a metabolic advantage over the other.[216]

In this study, 20 overweight adults were randomly assigned to one of two diets:

1. A ketogenic diet, consisting of 60% of calories from fats, 35% from protein, and 5% from carbohydrates

2. A traditional diet, consisting of 30% of calories from fats, 30% from protein, and 40% from carbohydrates

After 6 weeks, the results were as follows:

- There was no significant difference in total weight loss.

- Hunger ratings improved for both diets with no difference between them. This strikes at a claim often made to sell carb cycling, which is that it blunts hunger better than traditional dieting. According this study, that isn't true.

- Resting energy expenditure went up for both diets, with no difference between them. The low-carb diet failed to provide any special metabolic boost.

- Insulin sensitivity was improved in both diets, with no difference between them. This is yet another blow to the low-carb trend that's taking the fitness world by storm. The fact is weight loss in and of itself is effective at improving insulin sensitivity, regardless of diet composition.[217]

So, what you should take away from this section of the book is that the theory that low-carb days deliver the big fat loss punch of carb cycling are not supported by literature. They are simply part of the marketing pitch.

SOME ANECDOTAL SUPPORT FOR TRADITIONAL DIETING

I both advocate and use a traditional, flexible approach to dieting because it's simple, and it works very well when you do it right. The best diet is the one you can stick to, and you can get as lean as you want with traditional dieting.

I recently finished an 8 to 9-week cut using a traditional diet (40% of calories from protein, 40% from carbohydrates, and 20% from fats).

I lost about 13 pounds and went from ~9% down to ~6%, and my strength increased for the first 4 or 5 weeks and then decreased back to my pre-diet numbers over the course of the last several weeks (and this was simply because I had to gradually reduce my calories, and I chose to pull from carbs—this makes workouts harder).

Many other bodybuilders, fitness models, and fitness enthusiasts follow the same simple, traditional dietary protocol and get absolutely shredded. You do not have to do anything fancy with your diet to get lean.

Okay then, let's steam forward to the next big, bold claim made to sell people on carb cycling...

CAN YOU USE CARB CYCLING TO LOSE FAT AND BUILD MUSCLE SIMULTANEOUSLY?

The short answer?

Maybe.

But it's not the carb cycling per se that would make this possible. It would be your current level of conditioning, your training history, and your genetics.

For instance, I e-mail with scores of guys and gals every day who are losing fat and building muscle on my *BLS* and *Thinner Leaner*

Stronger programs, but they usually fit a certain profile:

- They're pretty out of shape to begin with and have a fair amount of fat to lose.

- They haven't lifted weights before or haven't lifted properly, which is to say they've never focused on lifting heavy weights, compound lifts, progressive overload, etc. Or they were once in good shape and have muscle memory on their side.

- They never quite knew what they were doing with their diets. Most have simply tried eating "clean" but have never calculated, tracked, and manipulated calories and macronutrients properly.

Under those circumstances, I *expect* people to both lose fat and build muscle while following my programs. But I don't try to claim it's because of the magical quantum mechanics of my methods like some carb-cycling hucksters. It's simply because the body responds incredibly well to proper diet and training, especially in the beginning. Newbie gains are real and are a lot of fun.

But if you're an advanced lifter who is approaching your genetic potential, I can guarantee you that you will not build muscle while losing fat without steroids, regardless of what you do in the kitchen or gym.

However, what you can and should strive for is maintaining the muscle you have by never putting yourself into too deep of a calorie deficit and not going overboard with too much steady-state cardio.

Another aspect of the carb cycler's claims of metabolic advantage is that your high-carb day will give your body an anabolic, muscle-building boost while simultaneously "shocking" your metabolism into high-gear, thus accelerating fat loss.

As you probably expect by now, these claims aren't supported by science.

I mentioned earlier that insulin can help preserve lean mass but does not induce muscle growth, and any metabolic boost that comes with increased caloric intake is offset by the extra calories themselves.[218][219] That is, you can speed your metabolism up by eating more but never to a point where you're burning the extra calories consumed plus additional fat.

Also relevant to this claim is the fact that most people get very stressed out on their no/low-carb days. If you want to know what carb cravings are like, eat fewer than 50 grams of carbs per day for a few days.

Training on a no/low-carb diet is even worse, and one or two higher carb days are not enough to offset this. If you want to drag ass and have basically the worst workouts ever, try to lift with any intensity following a couple of no/low-carb days.

Furthermore, a big part of maintaining lean mass while cutting is continuing to lift heavy weights and maintaining your strength, and drastic reductions in carbs make this impossible.

DOES CARB CYCLING HAVE ANY LEGITIMATE USES?

I've been pretty hard on carb cycling so far, but there are two particular circumstances where many people in the know use carb cycling and where I would consider it as well:

1. If you're looking to get really lean (under 7% body fat), then carb cycling may be able to help.

    While it may or may not inherently speed up fat loss, it can make maintaining a weekly calorie deficit easier for some. When you carb cycle, some days are higher calorie than others, but the weekly deficit is ultimately what matters (as you know). Some people enjoy eating less on their off days (they usually make these their low/no-carb days) and then being able to eat more on their training days, not unlike the surplus/deficit approach I outlined earlier in the book.

2. If you're looking to stay really lean (7% or under), carb cycling may also be able to help.

    For the same reasons stated above, many bodybuilders and fitness competitors use carb cycling to stay in contest shape for a couple of months out of the year while they're doing shows. It just makes it easier and more enjoyable for them to keep weekly caloric intake levels where they need to be.

Another benefit related to this point is that you will hold a little less subcutaneous (under the skin) water when you're carb cycling, thus making you look leaner.

HOW TO CARB CYCLE

There are many different systems for carb cycling out there, and I want to share with you a relatively simple cycle that you can use if you want to give carb cycling a try.

The cycle will involve rotating between two days:

- A high-carb day

- A low-carb day

Some methods include a day with fewer than 30 grams of carbohydrate intake, but this makes compliance even harder in exchange for few practical benefits.

You can use carb cycling to lose fat or to maintain a very low level of body fat percentage (5 to 7%). Let's look at both of these things separately.

HOW TO USE CARB CYCLING TO LOSE FAT

When you're carb cycling to lose fat, you will have three low-carb days followed by one high-carb day. Where you place your high-carb day doesn't matter much because it moves around week to week.

- For example, here's how it would look for me:

- Monday: Low-carb day

- Tuesday: Low-carb day

- Wednesday: Low-carb day

- Thursday: High-carb day

- Friday: Low-carb day

- Saturday (weak point training): Low-carb day

- Sunday (no weightlifting): Low-carb day

- Monday: High-carb day

- Tuesday: Low-carb day

- Wednesday: Low-carb day

- Thursday: Low-carb day

- Friday: High-carb day

- Saturday (weak point training): Low-carb day

- Sunday (no weightlifting): Low-carb day

- Monday: Low-carb day

- Tuesday: High-carb day

- And so forth.

Now, contrary to how carb cycling is often sold, you still have to plan and track your calorie/macronutritional intake if you want to guarantee results. If you don't, you will likely eat too much or too little, which can cause obvious problems (especially when you're trying to get really lean).

The starting point for proper calorie planning is your TDEE, which you calculate as discussed earlier in the book. As you know, fat loss requires a calorie deficit, and when you carb cycle, this deficit is larger on your low-carb days than your high-carb days.

On your low-carb days, set your calorie deficit at 20%, and on your high-carb days, set it at 10%. For example, my TDEE is about 2,800 calories per day, so my low-carb day's calories would be around 2,200, and my high-carb day's calories would be around 2,500.

Let's now look at how those calories translate into macronutrients.

- Your protein intake should always remain at 1 gram per pound of body weight.

- Your high-carb day consists of getting 50% of your daily calories from carbohydrates.

- Your low-carb day consists of getting 20% of your daily calories from carbohydrates.

- Your fat intake provides the rest of your calories (what's left after working out protein and carbohydrate intake).

Let's continue with my earlier TDEE calculation. Assume I am starting my cut at about 190 pounds. Thus, my high-carb day would look like this:

- 190 grams of protein

- 310 grams of carbs

- 55 grams of fat

And my low-carb day would look like this:

- 190 grams of protein

- 110 grams of carbs

- 110 grams of fat

I would then create a meal plan for both days and stick to them, alternating according to the 3:1 pattern. And in terms of meal planning, it's worth mentioning that the quality of the carbohydrates you eat matters a lot when you're carb cycling. Carb cycling is not well-suited for the "If It Fits Your Macros" types who want to eat junk carbs while trying to get and stay lean because it will lead to nutrient deficiencies.

To provide your body with the fiber and vitamins it needs to maintain optimal health, you should be getting all of your carbs from fruits, vegetables, unprocessed whole grains, and legumes.

The quality of the fats you eat matters as well. Make sure you get a balance of saturated and unsaturated fats.

HOW TO USE CARB CYCLING TO STAY LEAN

As with carb cycling for fat loss, there are various types of methods for carb cycling for maintenance, but the method I recommend is a 3:2 ratio (every five-day cycle consists of three low-carb days and two high-carb days).

The low-carb days help reduce water retention, making you look leaner, and the additional high-carb day is helpful for maintaining training intensity.

How you actually lay out the high- and low-carb days is up to you. Some people like to follow three low-carb days with two high-carb days, and others like to stagger them based on how they're feeling in the gym.

In terms of working out your numbers for your high- and low-carb days, you have two choices: you can maintain a level caloric intake every day (your TDEE) and just manipulate macronutrients, or you can eat a bit more on training days and a bit less on rest days (as discussed earlier).

As you know, I prefer the latter, but the former works as well. Either way, once you know how many calories you need to eat per day, here's how you work out the macronutrients:

- Your protein intake should always remain at 1 gram per pound of body weight.

- Your high-carb day consists of getting 40% of your daily calories from carbohydrates.

- Your low-carb day consists of getting 25% of your daily calories from carbohydrates.

- Your fat intake accounts for the rest of your calories (what's left after working out protein and carbohydrate intake).

I recommend that you schedule most of your high-carb days to fall on days you're lifting weights and most of your low-carb days on days you're not (although some of your training days will inevitably be low-carb days).

"F&*#AROUNDITIS" AND THE BIGGER PICTURE

Before we move on, I want to talk briefly about what Martin Berkhan (of LeanGains.com fame) called "f&*#arounditis." (Well, he was more explicit.) If we want to be more politically correct, we can call it Shiny Object Syndrome.

That is, too many people are looking for magic bullets, quick fixes, advanced body hacks, and other nonsense to reach their goals. One week they're following the Rebel Max Anabolic Anaconda Program, the next the X-Physique Metabolic Recomposition Program, and on, and on.

I have sympathy, but they're basically the hipsters of the lifting community. They're drawn to whatever is trending—whatever's buzzworthy. And they're always stuck in a rut.

I get e-mailed every day by people afflicted with Shiny Object Syndrome. It usually goes something like this:

Hey Mike,

I'm currently following an intermittent fasting protocol combined with some carb cycling and backloading. In the gym, I'm training twice per day on a power/hypertrophy triple-split, and I'm periodizing with German Volume Training. Why am I not big and lean like you? What type of cutting-edge protocols do you follow?

My reply usually leaves them a little baffled. I share my secrets:

- I lift heavy weights 5 to 6 times per week. I'm currently following the program in this book and am making great gains.

- I stick mainly to compound movements like the Squat, Deadlift, Bench Press, and Military Press. My isolation work is simply to prevent physique imbalances (Side and Rear Lateral Raises, and arms training).

- I always push myself to beat last week's numbers, even if it's only by one rep. Progressive overload is key.

- I eat a lot of protein and carbohydrates and enough fats to maintain health. If I want to lose fat, I put myself in a mild caloric deficit. If I want to maintain my body fat percentage, I eat (more or less) what I burn every day or week. And if I want to focus on building muscle, I put myself in a mild caloric surplus. My meal plan fits my dietary needs, schedule, lifestyle, and food preferences, and I stick to it. Period.

- I stay patient. I'm not looking for overnight results. I'm looking for small, weekly or biweekly improvements that, in time, add up to big changes.

That's it. That's all it takes.

Resist the allure of shiny objects. Don't contract f&*#arounditis.

There are no true shortcuts in this world. The path to physical greatness is the tried-and-true foundation of hard work and sensible eating and various tweaks that you can make to gain an extra bit here and there.

Now we've checked carb cycling off the list. Next, I'd like to talk about the ever-popular trend of Paleo dieting.

22

THE DEFINITIVE GUIDE TO THE PALEO DIET

LIKE CROSSFIT AND INTERMITTENT FASTING, THE Paleo diet has taken the health and fitness world by storm.

And like CrossFit and IF, the Paleo diet also has some big promises to make good on if you're to listen to the hype.

According to its more fervent supporters, the Paleo diet is the ultimate way to eat. The commonly touted benefits are quite impressive:

- Rapid, easy weight loss without having to count calories

- High, balanced energy levels with no crashes

- No cravings for junk

- Better workouts

- Protection against various types of disease, like cardiovascular disease and diabetes

- Clearer skin and prettier hair and teeth

- Reduced allergies

- Improved sleep

In short, many gurus sell the Paleo diet as the ultimate "diet hack": a way to put the power of genetics on your side and positively alter how your genes express themselves.

And if you combine it with CrossFit? Well, have you ever wanted to be superhuman?

Jokes aside, can the Paleo diet deliver on these claims?

Let's find out.

WHAT IS THE PALEO DIET?

Paleo is a contraction of Paleolithic, which refers to the Paleolithic Era in history, a period from about 2.5 million to 10,000 years ago. During this period, humans grouped together into small, roaming societies and developed simple tools to hunt and fish with.

The idea behind the Paleo diet is to eat how our ancient ancestors did—a diet mainly consisting of fish, grass-fed meats, eggs, vegetables, fruit, fungi, roots, and nuts. That's why it's also called the caveman diet, the Stone Age diet, and the hunter-gatherer diet.

The foods excluded from the Paleo diet are grains, legumes (peanuts, various types of beans, and chickpeas), dairy products, potatoes, refined salt, refined sugar, and processed oils (trans fats, as well as refined vegetable oils like canola, safflower, and sunflower oil).

As you can see, it's an inherently high-protein, low-carbohydrate, high-fat diet and has you eating a ton of animals and animal products.

If that sets off alarm bells in your head, warning of impending heart attacks or worse, hold your horses. We're going to address the health aspects of the Paleo diet in a minute, but first, let's start with a quick review of its theoretical foundations.

WHY SHOULD WE EAT LIKE CAVEMEN?

That's the first question I wondered when I heard about the Paleo diet.

Who cares how our ancient ancestors ate?

Well, the Paleo enthusiast would reply, for millions of years (before the Age of the Big Mac), us humans were hunter-gatherers. We had no agriculture, grocery stores, or ways to store and process food. We had to eat nuts, wild plants, and fresh meats. And, he will proclaim, we were much healthier back then—no arthritis, no cancer, no osteoporosis, and no heart disease. Thus, he will conclude, we should eschew modern dietary habits and return to our roots.

Well, while ancient humans may not have been as healthy as some people think, the idea still has an immediate appeal.[220] With disease exploding over the last century, something is deeply wrong with how modern humans are living, and diet is a primary culprit.

But is a return to the Stone Age the answer?

Well, the first problem with the theory of the Paleo diet is the assumption that just because a dietary behavior or method of food processing is more recent, it's automatically worse than the ancestral model.

Our prehistoric forebears had one thing in mind every day: *survival*. They ate whatever they could get their hands on, including each other sometimes.[221] (Uh, is human flesh Paleo-approved?) The point is their food choices weren't always optimal, and if we were transported back to Paleolithic times, we would be smart to decline a dinner invitation.

Although it doesn't have much bearing on the actual dietary protocols themselves, I found it slightly ironic that the Paleolithic humans didn't follow the Paleo diet.

The historical angle of the Paleo diet is based on a set of findings by its founder, Dr. Loren Cordain, and other researchers, which proposes that humans were primarily hunter-gatherers, with an emphasis on the hunting, during the Paleolithic era.[222]

This paper is an important piece of the scientific underpinnings of the Paleo diet and, in turn, is based on the flawed Ethnographic Atlas, a database on many cultural aspects of 1,167 societies.[223]

Primate ecologist Katherine Milton wrote an insightful paper on the matter, and here are a few highlights:

- The sources of data for the Ethnographic Atlas are mostly from the twentieth century. We've since learned that some societies coded as hunter-gathers weren't exclusively hunter-gatherers.

- Some of the authors who helped compile the Atlas were sloppy in their data collection. Furthermore, most of the researchers were male, and much of the collection and processing done by women was likely misreported or underreported.

- The hunter-gatherers included in the Atlas were modern-day humans, not people living in the primitive conditions of our distant past. The wide variety of dietary behaviors seen don't fall into a nice pattern that we can emulate. Furthermore, most of the hunter-gatherer societies lived off vegetable foods—an emphasis on hunting was rare.[224]

These critiques have been borne out by other studies.

- A study conducted by the Max Planck Institute for Evolutionary Anthropology reported that the diet of our early human ancestors, dating from about 2 million years ago, consisted almost exclusively of leaves, fruit, wood, and bark—similar to chimpanzees today.[225]

- A study conducted by researchers at the University of Calgary found that the diet of ancient Africans (going back as far as 105,000 years) may have been based on the cereal grass sorghum.[226] (Remember, grains are a big no-no in Paleo ideology.)

- Research conducted by scientists at the Center for Advanced Study of Hominid Paleobiology shows that the European Neanderthals ate starchy grains nearly 44,000 years ago.[227]

- Researchers from the Italian Institute of Prehistory and Early History also found that grains were regularly eaten by our Paleolithic ancestors.[228] Their findings suggest that processing vegetables and starches, and possibly even grinding them into flour, goes back as far as 30,000 years in Europe.

So, while the "eat like our ancestors" pitch makes for good marketing, the reality is doing it doesn't equate to the Paleo diet as we know it.

Now, even if that strips the Paleo diet of a bit of its scientific legitimacy and luster, it doesn't mean it's not a healthy way to eat.

The new question, then, becomes, *Even if our ancient ancestors weren't "Paleo," is the diet worthwhile nonetheless?*

MAKING A CASE FOR THE PALEO DIET

Here's the premise of the Paleo diet, as stated by its founder, Dr.

Loren Cordain:

> "With readily available modern foods, The Paleo diet mimics the types of foods every single person on the planet ate prior to the Agricultural Revolution (a mere 333 generations ago). These foods (fresh fruits, vegetables, meats, and seafood) are high in the beneficial nutrients (soluble fiber, antioxidant vitamins, phytochemicals, omega-3 and monounsaturated fats, and low-glycemic carbohydrates) that promote good health and are low in the foods and nutrients (refined sugars and grains, trans fats, salt, high-glycemic carbohydrates, and processed foods) that frequently may cause weight gain, cardiovascular disease, diabetes, and numerous other health problems. The Paleo diet encourages dieters to replace dairy and grain products with fresh fruits and vegetables—foods that are more nutritious than whole grains or dairy products."[229]

Despite his revisionist version of how our ancestors ate, it seems like a pretty sensible way to eat, no?

"But wait!" You might be thinking. "Won't eating a bunch of saturated fat cause your heart to explode?"

No, it won't. The myth that saturated fat intake is associated with heart disease has been thoroughly debunked, yet it still lingers.[230]

The reality is quite a few good things can be said about following the Paleo diet:

- It's a high-protein diet, which is quite healthy.[231]

- It emphasizes lean and not fatty, meats, which is an effective way to control caloric intake and prevent an imbalance between omega-3 and omega-6 fatty acid intake.

- It also excludes processed meats, which pose health risks.[232]

- It includes a lot of nutritious veggies and fruits, which decrease the risk of various diseases, such as cardiovascular disease, stroke, type 2 diabetes, and cancer.[233 234 235]

- It emphasizes a higher intake of omega-3 fatty acids, which provides a wide variety of health benefits such as reduced blood pressure, improved cognitive function, and the reduced risk of kidney and cardiovascular disease, stroke, and metabolic syndrome.[236 237 238 239 240 241]

- It excludes added sugars, which function as empty calories. Diets high in added sugars are often deficient in various micronutrients, because the foods high in such sugars usually have little nutritious value.[242]

- It excludes high-glycemic carbohydrates, which, if eaten regularly and in large enough quantities, can increase the risk of cardiovascular disease and diabetes.[243]

- It excludes trans fats, which increase the risk of cardiovascular disease and induce insulin resistance.[244]

There's no question: the Paleo diet *is* a healthy way to eat and is supported by peer-reviewed literature.

A study conducted by researchers at the University of California found that compared to the subjects' normal (poor) dietary habits, the Paleo diet improved blood pressure, glucose tolerance, insulin sensitivity, and lipid profiles.[245]

Another study conducted by researchers at the University of Lund found that the Paleo diet was better for type 2 diabetics than a traditional diabetes diet in terms of improving glycemic control (the body's ability to regulate blood sugar levels) and cardiovascular risk factors.[246]

So, clearly the Paleo diet has its merits. But the problems with the Paleo diet begin when we dive deeper into its dogma.

THE PROBLEMS WITH PALEO

The first big problem with Paleo is the stance that one singular way of eating is superior to all others.

The longest living populations on the planet are the peoples of Okinawa, Japan; Sardinia, Italy; Nicoya, Costa Rica; Ikaria, Greece; and the Seventh Day Adventists in Loma Linda, California—the Blue Zones, as these geographical locations have been labeled.

These people are quite un-Paleo—they don't eat much animal food and instead live on starch-based diets. To quote an extensive review on their dietary patterns: "...dietary patterns associated with longevity emphasize fruits and vegetables and are reduced in saturated fat, meats, refined grains, sweets, and full-fat dairy products."[247]

Equally notable is the wide variation in other aspects of healthy diets, particularly macronutrient intake. Traditional Okinawan diets provide ≥ 90% of calories from carbohydrate (predominantly from vegetables), whereas the traditional Mediterranean diet provides > 40% of calories from fat, mostly monounsaturated and polyunsaturated fat.

The point is while it's tempting to conclude that the diets of Blue Zoners are the best way to achieve optimal health, it would be erroneous to do so. There are too many other non-dietary factors that contribute to longevity. The same can be said for the Paleo diet.

The second big problem with the Paleo ideology is not what it has you eat but what it has you avoid.

By following the Paleo diet strictly, you miss potential benefits from foods like dairy, legumes, and whole grains, and the reasons given for avoiding such foods are scientifically flawed.

For instance…

- Dairy products are a good source of calcium, protein, and vitamin D, potassium, magnesium, zinc, and several other vitamins. Research has shown that dairy can improve bone health, muscle mass and strength, and even weight management.[248 249 250]

  Now, lactose intolerance is fairly prevalent and people can get these nutrients in other ways, but for those who do fine with dairy, it's a highly nutritious food.

  It's worth noting that I'm concerned with the quality of run-of-the-mill dairy here in the States due to the poor health of many of the dairy cows and the artificial hormones many are given that find their way into the milk.[251 252]

  These issues aren't part of the Paleo argument against dairy, though, which is simply that our ancient ancestors didn't eat dairy, so neither should we.

- Whole grains have been shown to reduce inflammation in the body and decrease the risk of cardiovascular disease, type 2 diabetes, and cancer and even to reduce mortality.[253 254 255 256]

Paleo gurus will often say that whole grains damage the intestines, but there simply isn't any reliable, in vivo (in living organisms) research available to support these claims.

As with dairy, some people don't do well with grains, but a true gluten intolerance is much less common than Paleo gurus would have you believe. And refined grains are not a good replacement for whole grains as they lose many of their nutrients during processing,[257] and have been associated with increased inflammation in the body.[258]

But for those that do fine with whole grains, they are a great source of carbohydrate, various nutrients, and fiber.

• Non-soy legumes have been shown to decrease total and LDL ("bad") cholesterol levels. They're also a good source of protein, carbohydrate, and fiber.[259]

Paleo proponents often say you should avoid legumes because they believe our ancestors didn't eat them and because they contain antinutrients that interfere with nutrient absorption.

While legumes do contain these antinutrients, so do many other foods, and they are reduced by simple processing methods like soaking and cooking.[260 261]

The bottom line is antinutrients found in whole grains and legumes are not a problem unless your diet is devoid of nutritious foods and horribly imbalanced in terms of macronutrients. Yes, if you mostly eat uncooked whole grains and beans all day, you will have some problems. However, there's no research to indicate that such antinutrients are a problem at normal intake levels and as a part of a properly balanced diet.

As you can see, while Paleo's approved foods are quite all right, its blacklisted foods just don't make sense.

One last little point I would like to address is the claim that you can lose weight on the Paleo diet without having to count calories.

I've worked with scores of people who weren't losing weight on the

Paleo diet simply because they had no concept of how many calories they were eating. Eating a healthy, low-carb diet doesn't mean you automatically lose weight—you have to maintain a caloric deficit.

THE BOTTOM LINE

While its historical foundations are flawed, the Paleo diet has a lot going for it. It's a heck of a lot healthier than the average person's diet, and you can derive many health benefits from it.

The mistake many people make with Paleo is accepting its extremes, which simply aren't scientifically defensible.

I eat fairly Paleo, because I enjoy meats, fruits, and vegetables. I also enjoy grains like rice, quinoa, and whole-grain pasta and bread, as well as a bit of dairy and legumes here and there.

Unsurprisingly, some of the less dogmatic and better informed Paleo gurus like Mark Sisson advocate this 80/20 approach. That is, you mostly eat meats, veggies, fish, fruit, and nuts, but you include limited amounts of dairy, grains, legumes, and other non-Paleo foods as needed or desired.

So, that's the last dietary protocol that I'd like to review with you. I hope you've found them helpful. In the next chapter, I want to share with you some tips about how to stay on track when you're traveling, as this can be quite frustrating if you don't have a correct strategy worked out.

23

HOW TO STAY IN SHAPE WHEN YOU'RE TRAVELING

US FITNESS FOLKS HAVE A LOVE/hate relationship with traveling.

Business travel usually means hectic schedules with no time to eat, which often drives people into the drive-thrus.

No matter how great a vacation is, after a couple of weeks of no exercise and overeating, we just can't wait to get back into the gym and restore balance to our lives (and scales).

Well, what if I told you that you travel without gaining weight or losing your conditioning?

What I told you that you could do it without following a strict eating schedule?

What if I told you that you could do it while still eating large "cheat" meals every day?

And what if I told you that you could do it with or without a proper gym?

Sounds too good to be true, right?

Well, I used to travel quite a bit, and in this chapter, I'm going to share you with several training and dietary strategies you can employ to minimally maintain your physique while traveling or even continue making progress as usual.

Let's begin…

HOW TO KEEP YOUR DIET
RIGHT WHILE TRAVELING

When traveling, the biggest dietary hurdle is regulating our caloric intake every day.

Traveling usually means eating out a lot, and restaurant food almost always comes with way more calories than we realize, thanks to butter, oils, sugar, and other sources of hidden calories.

The large daily surplus of calories plus reduced exercise is a particularly bad combination for our physiques.

It can also be a challenge to keep tabs on where our calories are coming from in terms of protein, carbs, and fats.

If you're following a weightlifting program and accidentally drop your protein intake to, let's say, 10% of your daily calories and stop working out for a couple of weeks, you're very likely to lose muscle.

Fortunately, you can do several things to avoid these problems—and you can do them while still maintaining a flexible daily schedule.

ENSURE YOU GET ENOUGH PROTEIN EVERY DAY

Protein is your staple nutrient for maintaining your muscle—you have to make sure you're getting enough every day.

The easiest way to keep track of your intake is a diet app like MyFitnessPal, which will allow you to research and track the nutrition data of the food you're eating or thinking about eating throughout the day. This takes the guesswork out and helps you make better choices about what you're eating.

PLAN YOUR MEALS ACCORDING TO YOUR GOALS

Before you give any thought to meal planning while traveling, you have to ask yourself what you want to see happen with your body while you're gone.

Are you cutting and want to continue to lose weight?

Would you like to just maintain your weight while you're away?

Are you okay with gaining some weight but want to keep it minimal?

Your choices will dictate your meal planning.

If you're cutting and want to continue losing weight, the easiest way to do this is to keep your meal plans simple.

Eating out too much, even if it's at restaurants like Chipotle that give you a rough idea of how many calories are in each meal, is the easiest way to halt weight loss.

Instead, what I like to do is create a simple meal plan out of foods that I can pick up at a local grocery store or health food store like Whole Foods and that don't require cooking or preparation.

Here are some of my favorite choices:

- Greek yogurt

- Protein powder

- Rotisserie chicken

- Low-sodium lean deli meat

- Low-fat cottage cheese

- Almonds and almond butter

- Fruit

- Salad (buy salad dressing and packaged greens)

When you book your hotel, make sure you ask about the mini-fridge. The bigger the better.

Then, when you land, you simply head to the grocery store, pick up your food, throw it in the fridge, and you're good to go. Not exciting, but it gets the job done.

If you'd like to maintain your current weight, you can be more flexible with your meal planning.

The reason being is you simply get to eat more food every day, and you have more wiggle room when you're maintaining.

What I like to do in this case is have a couple of meals per day that are planned ahead (as when cutting—foods that I can track exactly) and a couple of meals per day that aren't.

For the unplanned meals, I always stick to relatively simple foods and dishes whose numbers I can estimate with some accuracy using MyFitnessPal.

This way, I may end some days a little over maintenance and some a little under, but the net result is no noticeable fat storage.

I try not to be in a large caloric surplus more than one or two days per week.

If you're fine with gaining some weight but want to keep it minimal, you still need to watch what you're eating.

As we've all experienced, eating one meal of delicious "cheat" food can quickly turn into an all-out binge that, when you're on vacation, can last for days. (Yup, I've done it before!)

I like to avoid this by doing the same thing as I would if I were eating for maintenance, but my daily calories are higher. I generally eat a couple of planned meals per day and a couple of unplanned meals that I still track with decent accuracy.

REDUCE MEAL FREQUENCY IF NECESSARY

While I enjoy eating 5 to 7 small meals per day, I will usually reduce my meal frequency when I'm traveling to allow for larger, more calorie-dense meals.

For instance, if I know that I won't have access to much food for a large chunk of a day, don't like what I'll have access to (fast food, for instance), or want to save calories for a large meal that is planned, here's how it might go:

8 AM

50 g protein
100 g carbs
20 g fat

12 PM

50 g protein
10 g carbs
10 g fat

4 PM

30 g protein

5 g carbs

5 g fat

9 PM

100 g protein

150 g carbs

60 g fat

USE INTERMITTENT FASTING TO HELP

This is related to the meal frequency tip but warrants its own section because it's very useful when you're on the road.

Intermittent fasting not only allows us to benefit from a reduced meal frequency, but it also helps reduce fat storage due to the fat-burning effects associated with fasting.

The protocol I like best is the Leangains method created and popularized by Martin Berkhan, which we discussed earlier.

It's important that you don't use IF as an excuse to grossly overeat, however. It cannot prevent fat storage if you're in a large caloric surplus every day.

Here's what an average vacation day for me might look like using the intermittent fasting diet:

9 AM

I wake up and have a 0-calorie drink like tea. I drink plenty of water throughout the morning but don't eat any food.

1 PM

I hit a restaurant and have a steak, bread, a baked potato with butter and cheese, and some pie for dessert.

I check MyFitnessPal and calculate that the entire meal contained roughly 80 grams of protein, 150 grams of carbs, and 40 grams of fat.

5 PM

I don't want to have to eat 100 grams of protein at dinner (about what I'll need to hit my required protein intake for the day), so I have about 60 grams of protein in a shake.

8 PM

Dinner comes around and I enjoy a meal similar to lunch: 60 grams of protein, 100 grams of carbs, and 50 grams of fat.

This ends my eating for the day right around maintenance calories, or maybe in a slight surplus, and I got to enjoy two large meals.

My fasting period now begins, and I won't eat again until between 12 and 1 PM the next day.

If you can handle the fasting periods, this is a great way to minimize fat storage while still enjoying good food and maintaining a very flexible eating schedule that doesn't get in the way of everyone's plans ("DROP EVERYTHING! I NEED TO FIND PROTEIN NOW OR I'LL GO CATABOLIC!").

It's also very useful for when you won't have good foods available to you for longer periods. I've skipped many airport breakfasts to just make it up later at lunch once I had landed.

WORKING OUT WHILE TRAVELING

Getting workouts in while on the road is easier than some people think. You have several workable options:

- Stay in a hotel near a local gym.

  I always try to do this when traveling for work. My workout times might vary, but I can almost always fit a workout in, even if it's at 11 PM. I may do this while traveling for vacation—it just depends on the circumstances.

- Use the hotel gym.

  I know, hotel gyms suck, but they're better than nothing. Because they normally have very light weights and machines as, your best bet will probably be a 30 to 45 minute whole-body routine that you can perform a few days per week.

- Work out in your hotel room.

  If you can't hit a gym for whatever reason, you can still do a decent job of maintaining your conditioning with in-room training.

A device that is particularly good for this is the TRX Training System. It allows you to do a wide variety of body weight exercises, it weighs less than 2 pounds, and all you need to set it up is a door.

Another option is a simple full-body circuit that you can perform every day. Here's one I like:

- Push-Ups to failure (Knee Push-Ups are fine for women, if necessary)

- Rest 60 seconds

- Pull-Ups or Chin-Ups to failure if you can do them (you will need a pull-up bar)

- Rest 60 seconds

- Squats for 30 seconds (one-legged if possible)

- Burpees for 30 seconds

- Mountain Climbers to failure

- Rest 90 seconds

- Crunches to failure

- Rest 60 seconds

- Start over with Push-Ups

You can get a pretty good workout with this in 20 to 30 minutes.

- Do high-intensity interval cardio.

  If you'd rather just take a break from the weights or resistance training, or if you have the time and inclination to do both, you can do a 20 to 30 minute session of high-intensity interval cardio to help burn off excess calories.

- Do a workout before a meal if possible.

  Training before a meal helps us stay on track because it depletes our body's glycogen stores . When this occurs, the body is primed to replenish these stores, and it uses carbohydrate you eat to do this.[263]

Here's the kicker though: your body will not store carbohydrate you eat as fat until you replenish your glycogen levels.[264] This is the "carb sink" discussed earlier in the book.

So, by depleting a percentage of your glycogen stores before eating, you can, in a sense, buy yourself some "free carbs" in the post-workout meal.

As you can see, staying on track while traveling isn't nearly as hopeless as many people think.

By using the above strategies, I've gone on vacations for as long as 3 weeks, enjoyed large meals every day, and came back at exactly the same weight and conditioning as when I left.

The last thing I'd like to talk about is related to workout supplements. You may have suspected that it's a shady industry, but it's far worse than you think, and I think something should be done about it...

24

LET'S BRING CHANGE TO THE WORKOUT SUPPLEMENT INDUSTRY

AS AN AUTHOR, MY MISSION IS to help educate people on how to safely build muscle, lose fat, and get healthy as quickly and effectively as possible.

This includes raising people's awareness on the dirty secrets of the workout supplement industry and how to avoid wasting valuable time and money buying useless supplements and following ineffective training programs and nutrition plans.

You see, the reality is the workout supplement industry is plagued by pseudoscience, ridiculous hype, misleading advertising and endorsements, products full of junk ingredients, the underdosing of key ingredients, and many other shenanigans.

I talk about this in *BLS*, but I want to revisit it here, and you'll see why in a minute.

As you probably know, most supplement companies produce cheap, junk products and try to dazzle you with ridiculous marketing claims, high-profile (and very expensive) endorsements, pseudo-scientific babble, fancy-sounding proprietary blends, and flashy packaging.

They do it all because they don't want you to realize a simple truth of this industry: supplements don't build great physiques. Dedication to proper training and nutrition does.

You see, the supplement companies are cashing in BIG on a little trick that your mind can play on you known as the *placebo effect*.

This is the scientifically proven fact that your simple belief in the effectiveness of a medicine or supplement can make it work. People have overcome every form of illness you can imagine, mental and physical, by taking substances they believed to have therapeutic value but didn't. I'm talking about things like treating cancer and diabetes, eliminating depression and anxiety, and lowering blood pressure and cholesterol levels by taking medically worthless substances that people believed were treatments for their problems.

Many guys believe that the shiny new bottle of "muscle-maximizing" pills will work and then they sometimes do "feel them working." This is despite the fact that the ingredients used have never been scientifically proven to do anything the company claims, or even worse, have been proven ineffective.

So, while workout supplements do not play a vital role in building muscle and losing fat, and many are a complete waste of money…the right ones can help.

The truth of the matter is there *are* safe, natural substances scientifically proven to deliver benefits such as increased strength, muscle endurance and growth, fat loss, and more.

As a part of my work, it's been my job to know what these substances are and find products with them that I can use and recommend to others.

It's been pretty hard to do, though.

THE WILD GOOSE CHASE FOR WORTHWHILE WORKOUT SUPPLEMENTS

I've lived the fitness lifestyle for over a decade, have sold more than 200,000 books, and have helped thousands of people lose weight, build muscle, and get healthy.

For years now, I've been researching, testing, and recommending to others the best workout supplements I could find, but it was a constant struggle to maintain a list that met my standards.

What I've wanted for not just myself but others is simple:

- All ingredients backed by published scientific literature

- All dosages at clinically effective levels

- No artificial sweeteners, dyes, or unnecessary fillers

- Good taste

- Good value per serving

Apparently, that's way too much to ask, because these products simply haven't existed. Most don't even begin to come close to those standards. The egregious offenders of the workout supplement industry (of which there are many, unfortunately) do everything wrong:

- They use a ton of ingredients that have not been scientifically proven to do what is claimed.

- They underdose ingredients that actually work and use the proprietary blend to hide it.

- They stuff their products full of cheap chemicals and additives.

- They charge an arm and a leg.

So I did what I could. I found the best possible products for me and my readers, but in the back of my mind, I knew things could be done better.

As my career as an author began to grow and my tribe at my blog, Muscle for Life, began to form, I finally saw an opportunity to do something about the status quo that I hated so much.

I decided to take matters into my own hands and, I believe, add real value to the marketplace.

THE BIRTH OF LEGION

I created LEGION with a simple concept in mind: a supplement company dedicated to creating healthy, high-quality sport supplements based on sound science and dedicated to selling them honestly.

Furthermore, I want to create supplements that set the standard by which all others are judged, and I want to help educate consumers on the science of athletic performance so they can make better decisions in both their workout supplementation and training.

You see, I believe that you, as a consumer, are smarter than the industry elites give you credit for.

- I think you know dubious, or even fraudulent, marketing

claims when you see them.

- I think you question how effective a product can be if it contains tiny dosages of 67 different ingredients.

- I think you don't buy into A-list endorsements that are all about million-dollar paydays, not the products.

- I think you do care what you're putting into your body and want to know that the ingredients used are scientifically proven to be healthy, safe, and effective.

And so I decided that LEGION had to take a unique stand. It had to do what nobody else seemed to be willing to do:

NO PROPRIETARY BLENDS

There's absolutely no reason to use them for anything other than deception and fraud.

All the science behind effective ingredients and dosages is publicly available. Everyone knows what works and doesn't, and in what amounts. Claims of trade secrets are bogus.

If a company isn't willing to tell you exactly what you're buying, it's because it doesn't want you to know. Don't support these companies. Force them to change their ways.

At LEGION, we are 100% transparent about what's in our products and in what dosages. Not only that, but we also back each ingredient with scientific studies that you can review. When you buy a LEGION product, you know exactly what you're getting and why.

NO MISLEADING USE OF SCIENCE

Many workout supplement companies cite scientific studies to back up marketing claims because it works. An appeal to science is the easiest way to give your product an air of legitimacy.

But they're counting on something: that you don't go and review their citations.

You see, if you take the time review to the studies cited, you'll often discover one or more of the following to be true:

- The study findings are exaggerated or misconstrued to seem more significant than they are. Considering how much technical jargon is used in scientific literature, it's very easy to do this convincingly.

- The studies don't demonstrate the benefits at all. In fact, some studies cited actually demonstrate ingredients to be ineffective, yet they're cited as grounds for use.

- The subjects of the studies are elderly or diseased, not healthy adults. Just because a substance improves a sick person's condition in some way does not mean it will have the same effects in your body.

- The studies are animal research, not human research. While certain aspects of the human body share similarities with animals like pigs and rats, they are not similar enough to extrapolate animal research directly to humans. Animal research points the way for human research.

The marketing departments of the supplement companies that do these things know that the vast majority of consumers won't ever check their claims and don't know how to even if it occurred to them.

At LEGION, we rely only on scientific research that actually applies to our consumers, healthy adults who engage in regular exercise, and we are very careful to not exaggerate findings or make unfounded marketing claims.

NO LABEL-FILLER INGREDIENTS

A common practice in this industry is using a bunch of cheap ingredients that have no scientific backing and simply pad the ingredients list. This is done to make it seem like you're getting a lot for your money.

At LEGION, we use no label fillers. We have a simple standard that we live by: every active ingredient we use must be backed by published scientific literature that demonstrates clear performance benefits.

NO UNDERDOSING KEY INGREDIENTS

Most supplement companies have a simple problem: if you want to stick to using ingredients that have scientifically proven performance benefits, and if you want to use the same dosages as the studies proving their benefits…it gets expensive, fast.

That means less profit per sale and thus less money to spend on fancy marketing campaigns and endorsements.

So, what do the companies do instead?

They reduce manufacturing costs by using label-filler ingredients and by using tiny dosages of key ingredients (the ones backed by actual science).

When you compare other companies' dosages to the clinically effective dosages found in scientific studies, you quickly see the problem: they're a mere fraction of what scientists used to produce performance benefits.

Most companies hide this fact by using the proprietary blend and rely on their marketers to oversell the formulation.

At LEGION, we only use ingredients that we can include at clinically effective dosages: that is, the exact dosages shown to be safe and effective in published scientific research.

It makes our job harder, and we won't make nearly as much profit per sale as the "big boys," but we believe our products will represent a standard by which all others can be judged. And that matters most to us.

NO ARTIFICIAL SWEETENERS.

While artificial sweeteners may not be as dangerous as some people claim, studies suggest that regular consumption of these chemicals may indeed be harmful to our health and that more research is needed.[265,266,267,268] At LEGION, we've chosen to stay on the safe side and use the natural sweetener stevia instead.

Stevia is a plant with sweet leaves, and research has shown that it increases insulin sensitivity, helps regulate blood glucose levels, has anti-carcinogenic properties, decreases oxidative stress associated with eating large amounts of carbohydrates, reduces blood pressure and inflammation in the body, lowers bad cholesterol levels, and protects the kidneys.[269 270 271 272]

And in case you're worried that naturally sweetened means it tastes horrible, you can rest easy. We've taken special care to ensure that all of our products taste great, mix well, and go down easy.

NO ARTIFICIAL FOOD DYES.

Many supplements contain artificial dyes, known as azo dyes, such as FD&C Yellow #5, FD&C Blue #1, FD&C Red No. 40, and others.

Like artificial sweeteners, consumption of azo dyes might not be as harmful as some claim, but there is evidence that these chemicals can cause various negative effects in the body.[273 274 275 276 277]

At LEGION, we never use artificial food dyes because they carry potential health risks and add nothing but color. Do you care whether your pre-workout drink is a natural shade of light red or a deep, toxic-looking crimson?

I didn't think so.

NO EXAGGERATED, DECEPTIVE ADVERTISING OR ENDORSEMENTS.

Call us melodramatic, but we feel like we're getting slapped in the face every time we flip through a bodybuilding magazine.

Ad after ad features hulking freaks hawking one pill or powder or the other as if it has anything to do with why they're so big and lean.

How dumb do these marketers think we are?

At LEGION, we feel the facts alone should sell our products. Fitness models who truly believe in and endorse certain products are well and good, but that's of secondary importance.

NO OVERCHARGING AND UNDERDELIVERING.

How annoying is it to buy a $50 bottle of product only to discover that it only lasts 10 days if you follow the usage directions?

Half-filled buckets…ridiculously large serving sizes…recommendations of several scoops per serving.

We understand, and we disagree.

Because of our commitment to using clinically effective dosages and safe, healthy ingredients, we could price our products at the top of the market.

However, at LEGION, we not only provide you with—in some cases—4 to 5 times the effective ingredients per serving as our competitors, but we also ensure that you get enough in every bottle to last longer than a week or two.

THE HEART OF LEGION

We're committed to delivering effective workout supplements with high-quality, healthy ingredients that have published scientific literature to back them up and to providing a great value in terms of price and cost per serving.

You'll be hard pressed to find another sport supplement company as committed to good science, proper dosing, and healthy ingredients as we are. (I can save you the time and let you know that nobody else is doing it.)

I don't see us as just a supplement company. We're a research company.

We're obsessed with the world of health and fitness science and with educating ourselves and others on how we can safely and inexpensively optimize our athletic performance and thus get the most out of our training, sporting, and nutrition.

We're not just looking to build a company. We're looking to build a culture.

We believe in respecting our customers, telling things like it is, and delivering what we promise. We believe that honesty and integrity sell better than cutting corners and relying on ridiculous advertisements and lies.

We don't just want to sell you pills and powders; we want to change the supplement industry for the better.

Check us out at www.legionsupplements.com. I'd love to hear what you think.

25

THE ROAD AHEAD

WELL, WE'VE COME TO END OF this book but the beginning of a new chapter in your fitness journey.

If you put this book into use, you will have no problem building and maintaining a competition-worthy physique—lean, aesthetically proportionate, and healthy—and elite-level strength. And more importantly, you'll be able to do these things without making your entire life revolve around it, and you'll be able to enjoy them for the rest of your life.

As you'll see, these lofty goals don't require huge commitments of time in or out of the gym, extraordinary wisdom or genetics, or chemical enhancement. They only require doing a bunch of little things right, week in and week out, and patience.

My goal is to help you reach those goals, and I hope this book helps.

I want you to not only stay in shape but also to love your training just as much as when you started and to strive for a physique and level of strength that you used to think impossible. I want you to know that *anyone* can achieve superhuman levels of fitness.

If we work together as a team, we can and will succeed.

So, I'd like you to make a promise as you begin your transformation: Can you promise me—and yourself—that you'll let me know when you've reached your goal?

FREE BONUS REPORT: THE BEYOND BIGGER LEANER STRONGER CHALLENGE

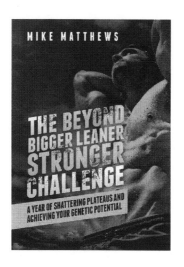

If you're ready to start the *Beyond Bigger Leaner Stronger* program, then you want to download this free bonus report.

Inside you'll find...

- An entire year's worth of *Beyond Bigger Leaner Stronger* workouts with links to videos showing proper form for all exercises.

- My latest product recommendations for supplements, workout equipment, kitchenware, books, and more.

- The definitive answer to whether you should cut or bulk first, and how to "juggle" these approaches properly for maximum gains.

- Examples of meal plans we create for people that want to build muscle and lose fat.

- Some of the most popular recipes from my bestselling cookbooks *The Shredded Chef* and *Eat Green Get Lean*.

- And more…

Download this free bonus report now and let's start shattering plateaus and setting new PRs!

VISIT HTTP://BIT.LY/BBLS-BONUS TO GET THIS REPORT NOW!

WOULD YOU DO ME A FAVOR?

Thank you for buying my book. I'm positive that if you just follow what you've learned, you'll shatter plateaus and achieve more in your workouts than you ever have before.

I have a small favor to ask. Would you mind taking a minute to write a blurb on Amazon about this book? I check all my reviews and love to get feedback (that's the real pay for my work—knowing that I'm helping people).

You can leave me a review by visiting the following URL:

www.bit.ly/bbls-review

Also, if you have any friends or family that might enjoy this book, spread the wisdom and lend it to them!

Now, I don't just want to sell you a book—I want to see you use what you've learned to build the body of your dreams.

As you work toward your goals, however, you'll probably have questions or run into some difficulties. I'd like to be able to help you with these, so let's connect up! I don't charge for the help, of course, and I answer questions from readers every day.

Facebook: facebook.com/muscleforlifefitness

Twitter: @muscleforlife

Instagram: instagram.com/muscleforlifefitness

G+: plus.google.com/+MikeMatthews

And last but not least, my website is www.muscleforlife.com and if you want to write me, my email address is mike@muscleforlife. com. (Keep in mind I get a lot of emails every day, and answer everything personally, so if you can keep yours as brief as possible, it helps me ensure everyone gets helped!)

Thanks again, I hope to hear from you, and I wish you the best!

Mike

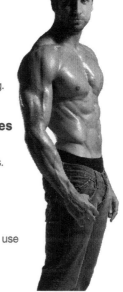

ALSO BY MICHAEL MATTHEWS

VISIT WWW.MUSCLEFORLIFE.COM TO LEARN MORE
ABOUT THESE BOOKS!

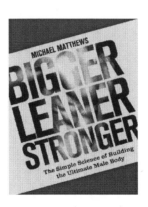

*Bigger Leaner Stronger: The Simple Science of Building the Ultimate
Male Body*

If you want to be muscular, lean, and strong as quickly as possible
without steroids, good genetics, or wasting ridiculous amounts of time
in the gym and money on supplements...then you want to read this
book.

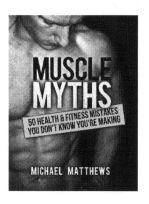

Muscle Myths: 50 Health & Fitness Mistakes You Don't Know You're Making

If you've ever felt lost in the sea of contradictory training and diet advice out there and you just want to know once and for all what works and what doesn't—what's scientifically true and what's false—when it comes to building muscle and getting ripped, then you need to read this book.

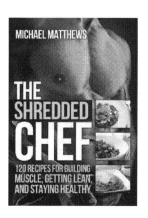

The Shredded Chef: 120 Recipes for Building Muscle, Getting Lean, and Staying Healthy

If you want to know how to forever escape the dreadful experience of "dieting" and learn how to cook nutritious, delicious meals that make building muscle and burning fat easy and enjoyable, then you need to read this book.

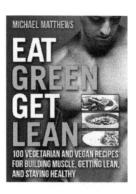

Eat Green Get Lean: 100 Vegetarian and Vegan Recipes for Building Muscle, Getting Lean and Staying Healthy

If you want to know how to build muscle and burn fat by eating delicious vegetarian and vegan meals that are easy to cook and easy on your wallet, then you want to read this book.

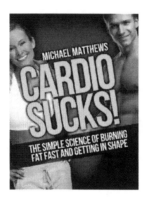

Cardio Sucks! The Simple Science of Burning Fat Fast and Getting in Shape

If you're short on time and sick of the same old boring cardio routine and want to kick your fat loss into high gear by working out less and...heaven forbid...actually have some fun...then you want to read this new book.

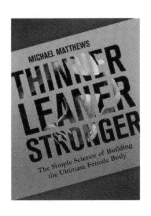

Thinner Leaner Stronger: The Simple Science of Building the Ultimate Female Body

If you want to be toned, lean, and strong as quickly as possible without crash dieting, "good genetics," or wasting ridiculous amounts of time in the gym and money on supplements...regardless of your age... then you want to read this book.

REFERENCES

1.   Neal, David T., Wendy Wood, and Jeffrey M. Quinn. "Habits—A repeat performance." Current Directions in Psychological Science 15, no. 4 (2006): 198-202.

2.   Lally, Phillippa, Cornelia HM Van Jaarsveld, Henry WW Potts, and Jane Wardle. "How are habits formed: Modelling habit formation in the real world."European Journal of Social Psychology 40, no. 6 (2010): 998-1009.

3.   Antonio, Jose. "Nonuniform Response of Skeletal Muscle to Heavy Resistance Training: Can Bodybuilders Induce Regional Muscle Hypertrophy?" The Journal of Strength & Conditioning Research 14, no. 1 (2000): 102-113.

4.   Ibid

5.   Per-Olof Åstrand, Kaare Rodahl, Hans A. Dahl, and Sigmund B. Strømme. Textbook of Work Physiology, 4th ed. (Champaign, IL: Human Kinetics, 2003), 56-59.

6.   A. Nardone, Carlo Romanò, and Marco Schieppati. "Selective Recruitment of High-Threshold Human Motor Units During Voluntary Isotonic Lengthening of Active Muscles," The Journal of Physiology 409 (1989): 451-71.

7.   Brad J. Schoenfeld. "The Mechanisms of Muscle Hypertrophy and Their Application to Resistance Training," Journal of Strength 24, no. 10 (2010): 2857-2872. doi: 10.1519/JSC.0b013e3181e840f3.

8.   Alfred L. Goldberg, Joseph D. Etlinger, David F. Goldspink, and Charles Jablecki. "Mechanism of Work-Induced Hypertrophy of Skeletal Muscle, Medicine and Science in Sports 7, no. 3 (1975): 185-198.

9.   Nicholas A. Burd, Cameron J. Mitchell, Tyler A. Churchward-Venne, and Stuart M. Phillips. "Bigger Weights May Not Beget Bigger Muscles: Evidence From Acute Muscle Protein Synthetic Responses after Resistance Exercise," Applied Physiology, Nutrition, and Metabolism 37, no. 3 (2012): 551-554. doi: 10.1139/h2012-022.

10. Phil J. Atherton and Ken Smith. "Muscle Protein Synthesis in Response to Nutrition and Exercise," Journal of Physiology 590 (2012): 1049-1057. doi:10.1113/jphysiol.2011.225003. http://jp.physoc.org/content/590/5/1049.full.

11. Vinod Kumar, Anna Selby, Debbie Rankin, Rekha Patel, Philip Atherton, Wulf Hildebrandt, John Williams, Kenneth Smith, Olivier Seynnes, Natalie Hiscock, and Michael J. Rennie. "Age-Related Differences in the Dose-Response Relationship of Muscle Protein Synthesis to Resistance Exercise in Young and Old Men," Journal of Physiology 587 (2009): 211-217. doi: 10.1113/jphysiol.2008.164483.

12. Nicholas A. Burd, Richard J. Andrews, Daniel W. D. West, Jonathan P. Little, Andrew J. R. Cochran, Amy J. Hector, Joshua G. A. Cashaback, Martin J. Gibala, James R. Potvin,

Steven K. Baker, and Stuart M. Phillips. "Muscle Time Under Tension During Resistance Exercise Stimulates Differential Muscle Protein Sub-Fractional Synthetic Responses in Men," Journal of Physiology 590 (2011): 351-362. doi: 10.1113/jphysiol.2011.221200.

13. Jeffrey J. Widrick, Julian E. Stelzer, Todd C. Shoepe, and Dena P. Garner. "Functional Properties of Human Muscle Fibers after Short-Term Resistance Exercise Training," American Journal of Physiology: Regulatory, Integrative and Comparative Physiology 283, no. 2 (2002): 408-16.

14. Ibid.

15. K. Häkkinen, A. Pakarinen, M. Alen, H. Kauhanen, and P. V. Komi. "Neuromuscular and Hormonal Adaptations in Athletes to Strength Training in Two Years," European Journal of Applied Physiology 65, no. 6 (1988): 2406-2412.

16. A. Nardone, Carlo Romanò, and Marco Schieppati. "Selective Recruitment of High-Threshold Human Motor Units During Voluntary Isotonic Lengthening of Active Muscles," The Journal of Physiology 409 (1989): 451-71.

17. Ibid.

18. Mathias Wernborn, Jesper Augustsson, and Roland Thomeé. "The Influence of Frequency, Intensity, Volume and Mode of Strength Training on Whole Muscle Cross-Sectional Area in Humans," Sports Medicine 37, no. 3 (2007): 225-264.

19. Arazi, Hamid, and Abbas Asadi. "Effects of 8 Weeks Equal-Volume Resistance Training with Different Workout Frequency on Maximal Strength, Endurance and Body Composition." Int J Sports Sci Eng 5, no. 2 (2001): 112-118.

20. Candow, Darren G., and Darren G. Burke. "Effect of short-term equal-volume resistance training with different workout frequency on muscle mass and strength in untrained men and women." The Journal of Strength & Conditioning Research 21, no. 1 (2007): 204-207.

21. MacDougall, J. Duncan, Martin J. Gibala, Mark A. Tarnopolsky, Jay R. MacDonald, Stephen A. Interisano, and Kevin E. Yarasheski. "The time course for elevated muscle protein synthesis following heavy resistance exercise." Canadian journal of applied physiology 20, no. 4 (1995): 480-486.

22. MCLESTER, JOHN R., PHILLIP A. BISHOP, JOE SMITH, LANA WYERS, BARRY DALE, JOSEPH KOZUSKO, MARK RICHARDSON, MICHAEL E. NEVETT, and RICHARD LOMAX. "A Series of Studies---A Practical Protocol for Testing Muscular Endurance Recovery." The Journal of Strength & Conditioning Research 17, no. 2 (2003): 259-273.

23. Bishop, Phillip A., Eric Jones, and A. Krista Woods. "Recovery from training: A brief review: Brief review." The Journal of Strength & Conditioning Research 22, no. 3 (2008): 1015-1024.

24. Mujika, I. Ñ. I. G. O., and S. A. B. I. N. O. Padilla. "Scientific bases for precompetition tapering strategies." Medicine and Science in Sports and Exercise 35, no. 7 (2003): 1182-1187.

25. Bell, G. J., D. G. Syrotuik, K. Attwood, and H. A. Quinney. "Maintenance of strength gains while performing endurance training in oarswomen." Canadian Journal of Applied Physiology 18, no. 1 (1993): 104-115.

26. Bickel, C. Scott, James M. Cross, and Marcas M. Bamman. "Exercise dosing to retain resistance training adaptations in young and older adults." Med Sci Sports Exerc 43, no. 7 (2011): 1177-87.

27. Carroll, Timothy J., Peter J. Abernethy, Peter A. Logan, Margaret Barber, and Michael T. McEniery. "Resistance training frequency: strength and myosin heavy chain responses to two and three bouts per week." European journal of applied physiology and occupational physiology 78, no. 3 (1998): 270-275.

28. Braith, R. W., J. E. Graves, M. L. Pollock, S. L. Leggett, D. M. Carpenter, and A. B. Colvin. "Comparison of 2 vs 3 days/week of variable resistance training during 10-and 18-week programs." International journal of sports medicine 10, no. 06 (1989): 450-454.

29. Candow, Darren G., and Darren G. Burke. "Effect of short-term equal-volume resistance training with different workout frequency on muscle mass and strength in untrained men and women." The Journal of Strength & Conditioning Research 21, no. 1 (2007): 204-207.

30. DeVries, Herbert A. "Physiology of exercise for physical education and athletics." (1974).

31. Langevin, Helene M., Debbie Stevens-Tuttle, James R. Fox, Gary J. Badger, Nicole A. Bouffard, Martin H. Krag, Junru Wu, and Sharon M. Henry. "Ultrasound evidence of altered lumbar connective tissue structure in human subjects with chronic low back pain." BMC musculoskeletal disorders 10, no. 1 (2009): 151.

32. Schleip, Robert. "Fascial plasticity–a new neurobiological explanation: Part 1." Journal of Bodywork and movement therapies 7, no. 1 (2003): 11-19.

33. Miernik, Marta, Mieszko Wieckiewicz, Anna Paradowska, and Wlodzimierz Wieckiewicz. "Massage therapy in myofascial TMD pain management." Advances in clinical and experimental medicine: official organ Wroclaw Medical University 21, no. 5 (2011): 681-685.

34. Findley, Thomas, Hans Chaudhry, Antonio Stecco, and Max Roman. "Fascia research–A narrative review." Journal of bodywork and movement therapies 16, no. 1 (2012): 67-75.

35. MacDonald, Graham Z., Michael DH Penney, Michelle E. Mullaley, Amanda L. Cuconato, Corey DJ Drake, David G. Behm, and Duane C. Button. "An Acute Bout of Self-Myofascial Release Increases Range of Motion Without a Subsequent Decrease in Muscle Activation or Force." The Journal of Strength & Conditioning Research 27, no. 3 (2013): 812-821.

36. Pinto, Ronei S., Naiara Gomes, Régis Radaelli, Cíntia E. Botton, Lee E. Brown, and Martim Bottaro. "Effect of range of motion on muscle strength and thickness." The Journal of Strength & Conditioning Research 26, no. 8 (2012): 2140-2145.

37. Sullivan, Kathleen M., Dustin BJ Silvey, Duane C. Button, and David G. Behm. "ROLLER-MASSAGER APPLICATION TO THE HAMSTRINGS INCREASES SIT-AND-REACH RANGE OF MOTION WITHIN FIVE TO TEN SECONDS WITHOUT PERFORMANCE IMPAIRMENTS." International journal of sports physical therapy 8, no. 3 (2013): 228.

38. Okamoto, Takanobu, Mitsuhiko Masuhara, Komei Ikuta, Minoh Niina, and Takanobu Okamoto. "Acute Effects of Self-Myofascial Release Using a Foam Roller on." (2013).

39. MacDonald, Graham Z., Duane C. Button, Eric J. Drinkwater, and David George Behm. "Foam Rolling as a Recovery Tool after an Intense Bout of Physical Activity." Medicine & Science in Sports & Exercise 46, no. 1 (2014): 131-142.

40. Reilly, Thomas, and Mark Piercy. "The effect of partial sleep deprivation on weight-lifting performance." Ergonomics 37, no. 1 (1994): 107-115.

41. Samuels, Charles. "Sleep, recovery, and performance: the new frontier in high-performance athletics." Physical medicine and rehabilitation clinics of North America

20, no. 1 (2009): 149-159.

42. Mah, Cheri D., Kenneth E. Mah, Eric J. Kezirian, and William C. Dement. "The effects of sleep extension on the athletic performance of collegiate basketball players." Sleep 34, no. 7 (2011): 943.

43. http://www.nytimes.com/2011/04/17/magazine/mag-17Sleep-t.html?_r=0

44. Frøsig, Christian, and Erik A. Richter. "Improved insulin sensitivity after exercise: focus on insulin signaling." Obesity 17, no. S3 (2009): S15-S20.

45. Wang, Xiaonan, Zhaoyong Hu, Junping Hu, Jie Du, and William E. Mitch. "Insulin resistance accelerates muscle protein degradation: Activation of the ubiquitin-proteasome pathway by defects in muscle cell signaling." Endocrinology 147, no. 9 (2006): 4160-4168.

46. Wilson, Jacob M., Pedro J. Marin, Matthew R. Rhea, Stephanie MC Wilson, Jeremy P. Loenneke, and Jody C. Anderson. "Concurrent training: a meta-analysis examining interference of aerobic and resistance exercises." The Journal of Strength & Conditioning Research 26, no. 8 (2012): 2293-2307.

47. Marshall, Paul WM, Daniel A. Robbins, Anthony W. Wrightson, and Jason C. Siegler. "Acute neuromuscular and fatigue responses to the rest-pause method." Journal of Science and Medicine in Sport 15, no. 2 (2012): 153-158.

48. Johnstone, Alexandra M., Sandra D. Murison, Jackie S. Duncan, Kellie A. Rance, and John R. Speakman. "Factors influencing variation in basal metabolic rate include fat-free mass, fat mass, age, and circulating thyroxine but not sex, circulating leptin, or triiodothyronine." The American journal of clinical nutrition 82, no. 5 (2005): 941-948.

49. Mifflin, Mark D., S. T. St Jeor, Lisa A. Hill, Barbara J. Scott, Sandra A. Daugherty, and Y. O. Koh. "A new predictive equation for resting energy expenditure in healthy individuals." The American journal of clinical nutrition 51, no. 2 (1990): 241-247.

50. Speakman, John R., Elżbieta Król, and Maria S. Johnson. "The functional significance of individual variation in basal metabolic rate." Physiological and Biochemical Zoology 77, no. 6 (2004): 900-915.

51. Martin, Corby K., Leonie K. Heilbronn, Lilian Jonge, James P. DeLany, Julia Volaufova, Stephen D. Anton, Leanne M. Redman, Steven R. Smith, and Eric Ravussin. "Effect of calorie restriction on resting metabolic rate and spontaneous physical activity." Obesity 15, no. 12 (2007): 2964-2973.

52. Redman, Leanne M., Leonie K. Heilbronn, Corby K. Martin, Lilian de Jonge, Donald A. Williamson, James P. Delany, and Eric Ravussin. "Metabolic and behavioral compensations in response to caloric restriction: implications for the maintenance of weight loss." PLoS One 4, no. 2 (2009): e4377.

53. Harris, Ann M., Michael D. Jensen, and James A. Levine. "Weekly changes in basal metabolic rate with eight weeks of overfeeding." Obesity 14, no. 4 (2006): 690-695.

54. Dulloo, Abdul G., Jean Jacquet, and Jean-Pierre Montani. "Session II: Metabolic flexibility and regulation How dieting makes some fatter: from a perspective of human body composition autoregulation." Proceedings of the Nutrition Society(2012).

55. Fatouros, Ioannis G., Athanasios Chatzinikolaou, Symeon Tournis, Michalis G. Nikolaidis, Athanasios Z. Jamurtas, Ioannis I. Douroudos, Ioannis Papassotiriou et al. "Intensity of resistance exercise determines adipokine and resting energy expenditure responses in overweight elderly individuals." Diabetes care 32, no. 12 (2009): 2161-2167.

56. Wang, ZiMian, Stanley Heshka, Kuan Zhang, Carol N. Boozer, and Steven B. Heymsfield. "Resting Energy Expenditure: Systematic Organization and Critique of Prediction Methods&ast." Obesity 9, no. 5 (2001): 331-336.

57. Dorgan, Joanne F., Joseph T. Judd, Christopher Longcope, Charles Brown, Arthur Schatzkin, Beverly A. Clevidence, William S. Campbell et al. "Effects of dietary fat and fiber on plasma and urine androgens and estrogens in men: a controlled feeding study." The American journal of clinical nutrition 64, no. 6 (1996): 850-855.

58. Welle, S. T. E. P. H. E. N., R. A. L. P. H. Jozefowicz, G. I. L. B. E. R. T. Forbes, and ROBERT C. Griggs. "Effect of testosterone on metabolic rate and body composition in normal men and men with muscular dystrophy." The Journal of clinical endocrinology and metabolism 74, no. 2 (1992): 332-335.

59. Newsholme, E. A., and G. Dimitriadis. "Integration of biochemical and physiologic effects of insulin on glucose metabolism." Experimental and Clinical Endocrinology & Diabetes 109, no. Suppl 2 (2001): S122-S134.

60. Surina, D. M., W. Langhans, R. Pauli, and C. Wenk. "Meal composition affects postprandial fatty acid oxidation." American Journal of Physiology-Regulatory, Integrative and Comparative Physiology 264, no. 6 (1993): R1065-R1070.

61. LEFKOWITZ, ROBERT J. "Direct binding studies of adrenergic receptors: biochemical, physiologic, and clinical implications." Annals of internal Medicine 91, no. 3 (1979): 450-458.

62. Strosberg, A. D. "Structure, function, and regulation of adrenergic receptors." Protein Science 2, no. 8 (1993): 1198-1209.

63. Tomiyama, A. Janet, Traci Mann, Danielle Vinas, Jeffrey M. Hunger, Jill DeJager, and Shelley E. Taylor. "Low calorie dieting increases cortisol."Psychosomatic medicine 72, no. 4 (2010): 357-364.

64. Redman, Leanne M., Leonie K. Heilbronn, Corby K. Martin, Lilian De Jonge, Donald A. Williamson, James P. Delany, and Eric Ravussin. "Metabolic and behavioral compensations in response to caloric restriction: implications for the maintenance of weight loss." PLoS One 4, no. 2 (2009): e4377.

65. Durrant, Merril L., J. S. Garrow, P. Royston, Susan F. Stalley, Shirley Sunkin, and Penelope M. Warwick. "Factors influencing the composition of the weight lost by obese patients on a reducing diet." British journal of nutrition 44, no. 03 (1980): 275-285.

66. Cangemi, Roberto, Alberto J. Friedmann, John O. Holloszy, and Luigi Fontana. "Long-term effects of calorie restriction on serum sex-hormone concentrations in men." Aging cell 9, no. 2 (2010): 236-242.

67. Cribb, Paul J., and Alan Hayes. "Effects of Supplement-Timing and Resistance Exercise on Skeletal Muscle Hypertrophy." Medicine & Science in Sports & Exercise 38, no. 11 (2006): 1918-1925.

68. Ivy, J. L. "Glycogen resynthesis after exercise: effect of carbohydrate intake." International journal of sports medicine 19, no. 2 (1998): S142.

69. Howarth, Krista R., Stuart M. Phillips, Maureen J. MacDonald, Douglas Richards, Natalie A. Moreau, and Martin J. Gibala. "Effect of glycogen availability on human skeletal muscle protein turnover during exercise and recovery." Journal of Applied Physiology 109, no. 2 (2010): 431-438.

70. Levitsky, David A., and Carly R. Pacanowski. "Effect of skipping breakfast on subsequent

energy intake." Physiology & behavior 119 (2013): 9-16.

71. Redman, Leanne M., Leonie K. Heilbronn, Corby K. Martin, Lilian De Jonge, Donald A. Williamson, James P. Delany, and Eric Ravussin. "Metabolic and behavioral compensations in response to caloric restriction: implications for the maintenance of weight loss." PLoS One 4, no. 2 (2009): e4377.

72. Davis, Jon F., Derrick L. Choi, and Stephen C. Benoit. "Insulin, leptin and reward." Trends in Endocrinology & Metabolism 21, no. 2 (2010): 68-74.

73. Davis, Jon F. "Adipostatic regulation of motivation and emotion." Discovery medicine 9, no. 48 (2010): 462.

74. Hausman, G. J., and C. R. Barb. "Adipose tissue and the reproductive axis: biological aspects." (2010): 31-44.

75. Jéquier, Eric. "Leptin signaling, adiposity, and energy balance." Annals of the New York Academy of Sciences 967, no. 1 (2002): 379-388.

76. Ceddia, R. B. "Direct metabolic regulation in skeletal muscle and fat tissue by leptin: implications for glucose and fatty acids homeostasis." International journal of obesity 29, no. 10 (2005): 1175-1183.

77. Ahima, Rexford S., Daniel Prabakaran, Christos Mantzoros, Daqing Qu, Bradford Lowell, Eleftheria Maratos-Flier, and Jeffrey S. Flier. "Role of leptin in the neuroendocrine response to fasting." (1996): 250-252.

78. Lu, Xin-Yun. "The leptin hypothesis of depression: a potential link between mood disorders and obesity?." Current opinion in pharmacology 7, no. 6 (2007): 648-652.

79. Söderberg, S., T. Olsson, M. Eliasson, O. Johnson, K. Brismar, K. Carlström, and B. Ahren. "A strong association between biologically active testosterone and leptin in non-obese men and women is lost with increasing (central) adiposity." International Journal of Obesity & Related Metabolic Disorders 25, no. 1 (2001).

80. Dirlewanger, M., V. Di Vetta, E. Guenat, P. Battilana, G. Seematter, P. Schneiter, E. Jéquier, and L. Tappy. "Effects of short-term carbohydrate or fat overfeeding on energy expenditure and plasma leptin concentrations in healthy female subjects." International Journal of Obesity & Related Metabolic Disorders 24, no. 11 (2000).

81. Weigle, David S., Patricia A. Breen, Colleen C. Matthys, Holly S. Callahan, Kaatje E. Meeuws, Verna R. Burden, and Jonathan Q. Purnell. "A high-protein diet induces sustained reductions in appetite, ad libitum caloric intake, and body weight despite compensatory changes in diurnal plasma leptin and ghrelin concentrations." The American journal of clinical nutrition 82, no. 1 (2005): 41-48.

82. Dirlewanger, M., V. Di Vetta, E. Guenat, P. Battilana, G. Seematter, P. Schneiter, E. Jéquier, and L. Tappy. "Effects of short-term carbohydrate or fat overfeeding on energy expenditure and plasma leptin concentrations in healthy female subjects." International Journal of Obesity & Related Metabolic Disorders 24, no. 11 (2000).

83. Röjdmark, S., J. Calissendorff, and K. Brismar. "Alcohol ingestion decreases both diurnal and nocturnal secretion of leptin in healthy individuals." Clinical endocrinology 55, no. 5 (2001): 639-647.

84. Siri-Tarino, Patty W., Qi Sun, Frank B. Hu, and Ronald M. Krauss. "Meta-analysis of prospective cohort studies evaluating the association of saturated fat with cardiovascular disease." The American journal of clinical nutrition 91, no. 3 (2010): 535-546.

85. Mente, Andrew, Lawrence de Koning, Harry S. Shannon, and Sonia S. Anand. "A systematic review of the evidence supporting a causal link between dietary factors and coronary heart disease." Archives of internal medicine 169, no. 7 (2009): 659-669.

86. Horton, Tracy J., Holly Drougas, Amy Brachey, George W. Reed, John C. Peters, and J. O. Hill. "Fat and carbohydrate overfeeding in humans: different effects on energy storage." The American journal of clinical nutrition 62, no. 1 (1995): 19-29.

87. Tessari, Paolo, Sandro Inchiostro, Gianni Biolo, Ezio Vincenti, and Luigi Sabadin. "Effects of acute systemic hyperinsulinemia on forearm muscle proteolysis in healthy man." Journal of Clinical Investigation 88, no. 1 (1991): 27.

88. Holt, S. H., J. C. Miller, and Peter Petocz. "An insulin index of foods: the insulin demand generated by 1000-kJ portions of common foods." The American journal of clinical nutrition 66, no. 5 (1997): 1264-1276.

89. McDevitt, Regina M., Sarah J. Bott, Marilyn Harding, W. Andrew Coward, Leslie J. Bluck, and Andrew M. Prentice. "De novo lipogenesis during controlled overfeeding with sucrose or glucose in lean and obese women." The American journal of clinical nutrition 74, no. 6 (2001): 737-746.

90. Ibid.

91. Kreitzman, Stephen N., Ann Y. Coxon, and Kalman F. Szaz. "Glycogen storage: illusions of easy weight loss, excessive weight regain, and distortions in estimates of body composition." The American journal of clinical nutrition 56, no. 1 (1992): 292S-293S.

92. Olsson, Karl-Erik, and Bengt Saltin. "Variation in total body water with muscle glycogen changes in man." Acta Physiologica Scandinavica 80, no. 1 (1970): 11-18.

93. Ibid.

94. Kleiner, Rima E., Andrea M. Hutchins, Carol S. Johnston, and Pamela D. Swan. "Effects of an 8-week high-protein or high-carbohydrate diet in adults with hyperinsulinemia." Medscape General Medicine 8, no. 4 (2006): 39.

95. Dansinger, Michael L., Joi Augustin Gleason, John L. Griffith, Harry P. Selker, and Ernst J. Schaefer. "Comparison of the Atkins, Ornish, Weight Watchers, and Zone diets for weight loss and heart disease risk reduction: a randomized trial." Jama 293, no. 1 (2005): 43-53.

96. Blundell, John E., J. Cooling, and Neil A. King. "Differences in postprandial responses to fat and carbohydrate loads in habitual high and low fat consumers (phenotypes)." British Journal of Nutrition 88, no. 02 (2002): 125-132.

97. Cooling, J., and J. E. Blundell. "Lean male high-and low-fat phenotypes—different routes for achieving energy balance." International Journal of Obesity & Related Metabolic Disorders 24, no. 12 (2000).

98. Blundell, John E., and John Cooling. "High-fat and low-fat (behavioural) phenotypes: biology or environment?." Proceedings of the Nutrition Society 58, no. 04 (1999): 773-777.

99. Pittas, Anastassios G., and Susan B. Roberts. "Dietary composition and weight loss: can we individualize dietary prescriptions according to insulin sensitivity or secretion status?." Nutrition reviews 64, no. 10 (2006): 435-448.

100. A de Luis, D., R. Aller, O. Izaola, M. Gonzalez Sagrado, and R. Conde. "Differences in glycaemic status do not predict weight loss in response to hypocaloric diets in obese

patients." Clinical Nutrition 25, no. 1 (2006): 117-122.

101. Pittas, Anastassios G., Sai Krupa Das, Cheryl L. Hajduk, Julie Golden, Edward Saltzman, Paul C. Stark, Andrew S. Greenberg, and Susan B. Roberts. "A low-glycemic load diet facilitates greater weight loss in overweight adults with high insulin secretion but not in overweight adults with low insulin secretion in the CALERIE Trial." Diabetes Care 28, no. 12 (2005): 2939-2941.

102. Cornier, Marc-Andre, W. Troy Donahoo, Rocio Pereira, Inga Gurevich, Rickard Westergren, Sven Enerback, Peter J. Eckel et al. "Insulin sensitivity determines the effectiveness of dietary macronutrient composition on weight loss in obese women." Obesity research 13, no. 4 (2005): 703-709.

103. Cangemi, Roberto, Alberto J. Friedmann, John O. Holloszy, and Luigi Fontana. "Long-term effects of calorie restriction on serum sex-hormone concentrations in men." Aging cell 9, no. 2 (2010): 236-242.

104. Pasiakos, Stefan M., Lisa M. Vislocky, John W. Carbone, Nicholas Altieri, Karen Konopelski, Hedley C. Freake, Jeffrey M. Anderson, Arny A. Ferrando, Robert R. Wolfe, and Nancy R. Rodriguez. "Acute energy deprivation affects skeletal muscle protein synthesis and associated intracellular signaling proteins in physically active adults." The Journal of nutrition 140, no. 4 (2010): 745-751.

105. A. Janet Tomiyama, Traci Mann, Danielle Vinas, Jeffrey M. Hunger, Jill DeJager, and Shelley E. Taylor. "Low Calorie Dieting Increases Cortisol," Psychosomatic Medicine 72, no. 4: 357-64. doi: 10.1097/PSY.0b013e3181d9523c.

106. Tremblay, Angelo, Jean-Aimé Simoneau, and Claude Bouchard. "Impact of exercise intensity on body fatness and skeletal muscle metabolism."Metabolism 43, no. 7 (1994): 814-818.

107. King, Jeffrey W. "A comparison of the effects of interval training vs. continuous training on weight loss and body composition in obese pre-menopausal women." PhD diss., East Tennessee State University, 2001.

108. Treuth, MARGARITA S., GARY R. Hunter, and M. A. R. T. H. A. Williams. "Effects of exercise intensity on 24-h energy expenditure and substrate oxidation." Medicine and science in sports and exercise 28, no. 9 (1996): 1138.

109. Trapp, E. G., D. J. Chisholm, J. Freund, and S. H. Boutcher. "The effects of high-intensity intermittent exercise training on fat loss and fasting insulin levels of young women." International journal of obesity 32, no. 4 (2008): 684-691.

110. Macpherson, R. E., Tom J. Hazell, T. Dylan Olver, Don H. Paterson, and P. W. Lemon. "Run sprint interval training improves aerobic performance but not maximal cardiac output." Med Sci Sports Exerc 43, no. 1 (2011): 115-22.

111. Boutcher, Stephen H. "High-intensity intermittent exercise and fat loss." Journal of obesity 2011 (2010).

112. Gergley, Jeffrey C. "Comparison of two lower-body modes of endurance training on lower-body strength development while concurrently training." The Journal of Strength & Conditioning Research 23, no. 3 (2009): 979-987.

113. Moolyk, Amy N., Jason P. Carey, and Loren ZF Chiu. "Performance and Neuromuscular Adaptations Following Differing Ratios of Concurrent Strength and Endurance Training." Journal of Strength & Conditioning Research 27, no. 12 (2013): 3342-3351.

114. Gergley, Jeffrey C. "Comparison of two lower-body modes of endurance training on

lower-body strength development while concurrently training." The Journal of Strength & Conditioning Research 23, no. 3 (2009): 979-987.

115. Derave, Wim, Ann Mertens, Erik Muls, Karel Pardaens, and Peter Hespel. "Effects of Post-absorptive and Postprandial Exercise on Glucoregulation in Metabolic Syndrome." Obesity 15, no. 3 (2007): 704-711.

116. Achten, Juul, and Asker E. Jeukendrup. "Optimizing fat oxidation through exercise and diet." Nutrition 20, no. 7 (2004): 716-727.

117. Kraemer, William J., Steven J. Fleck, Carl M. Maresh, Nicholas A. Ratamess, Scott E. Gordon, Kenneth L. Goetz, Everett A. Harman et al. "Acute hormonal responses to a single bout of heavy resistance exercise in trained power lifters and untrained men." Canadian journal of applied physiology 24, no. 6 (1999): 524-537.

118. Deldicque, Louise, Katrien De Bock, Michael Maris, Monique Ramaekers, Henri Nielens, Marc Francaux, and Peter Hespel. "Increased p70s6k phosphorylation during intake of a protein–carbohydrate drink following resistance exercise in the fasted state." European journal of applied physiology 108, no. 4 (2010): 791-800.

119. Pitkanen, H. T., T. A. R. J. A. Nykanen, J. U. H. A. Knuutinen, K. A. I. S. A. Lahti, O. L. A. V. I. Keinanen, M. A. R. K. K. U. Alen, PAAVO V. Komi, and ANTTI A. Mero. "Free amino acid pool and muscle protein balance after resistance exercise." Medicine and science in sports and exercise 35, no. 5 (2003): 784-792.

120. Fujita, Satoshi, Hans C. Dreyer, Micah J. Drummond, Erin L. Glynn, Jerson G. Cadenas, Fumiaki Yoshizawa, Elena Volpi, and Blake B. Rasmussen. "Nutrient signalling in the regulation of human muscle protein synthesis." The Journal of physiology 582, no. 2 (2007): 813-823.

121. Howatson, Glyn, Michael Hoad, Stuart Goodall, Jamie Tallent, Phillip G. Bell, and Duncan N. French. "Exercise-induced muscle damage is reduced in resistance-trained males by branched chain amino acids: a randomized, double-blind, placebo controlled study." J Int Soc Sports Nutr 9, no. 1 (2012): 20.

122. Power, O., A. Hallihan, and P. Jakeman. "Human insulinotropic response to oral ingestion of native and hydrolysed whey protein." Amino acids 37, no. 2 (2009): 333-339.

123. Capaldo, Brunella, Amalia Gastaldelli, Salvatore Antoniello, Maria Auletta, Francesco Pardo, Demetrio Ciociaro, Raffaele Guida, Ele Ferrannini, and Luigi Saccà. "Splanchnic and leg substrate exchange after ingestion of a natural mixed meal in humans." Diabetes 48, no. 5 (1999): 958-966.

124. Choi, Sarah M., David F. Tucker, Danielle N. Gross, Rachael M. Easton, Lisa M. DiPilato, Abigail S. Dean, Bob R. Monks, and Morris J. Birnbaum. "Insulin regulates adipocyte lipolysis via an Akt-independent signaling pathway."Molecular and cellular biology 30, no. 21 (2010): 5009-5020.

125. Astorino, Todd A., Riana L. Rohmann, and Kelli Firth. "Effect of caffeine ingestion on one-repetition maximum muscular strength." European journal of applied physiology 102, no. 2 (2008): 127-132.

126. Beck, Travis W., Terry J. Housh, Richard J. Schmidt, Glen O. Johnson, Dona J. Housh, Jared W. Coburn, and Moh H. Malek. "The acute effects of a caffeine-containing supplement on strength, muscular endurance, and anaerobic capabilities." The Journal of Strength & Conditioning Research 20, no. 3 (2006): 506-510.

127. Ibid.

128. Mora-Rodríguez, Ricardo, Jesús García Pallarés, Álvaro López-Samanes, Juan Fernando Ortega, and Valentín E. Fernández-Elías. "Caffeine ingestion reverses the circadian rhythm effects on neuromuscular performance in highly resistance-trained men." PloS one 7, no. 4 (2012): e33807.

129. Astrup, A., S. Toubro, S. Cannon, P. Hein, L. Breum, and J. Madsen. "Caffeine: a double-blind, placebo-controlled study of its thermogenic, metabolic, and cardiovascular effects in healthy volunteers." The American journal of clinical nutrition 51, no. 5 (1990): 759-767.

130. Ibid.

131. LeBlanc, J. A. C. Q. U. E. S., M. I. C. H. E. L. Jobin, J. Cote, P. I. E. R. R. E. Samson, and A. N. T. O. I. N. E. Labrie. "Enhanced metabolic response to caffeine in exercise-trained human subjects." Journal of Applied Physiology 59, no. 3 (1985): 832-837.

132. Goldstein, Erica R., Tim Ziegenfuss, Doug Kalman, Richard Kreider, Bill Campbell, Colin Wilborn, Lem Taylor et al. "International society of sports nutrition position stand: caffeine and performance." J Int Soc Sports Nutr 7, no. 1 (2010): 5.

133. Yang, Chung S., Joshua D. Lambert, and Shengmin Sang. "Antioxidative and anti-carcinogenic activities of tea polyphenols." Archives of toxicology 83, no. 1 (2009): 11-21.

134. Venables, Michelle C., Carl J. Hulston, Hannah R. Cox, and Asker E. Jeukendrup. "Green tea extract ingestion, fat oxidation, and glucose tolerance in healthy humans." The American journal of clinical nutrition 87, no. 3 (2008): 778-784.

135. Maki, Kevin C., Matthew S. Reeves, Mildred Farmer, Koichi Yasunaga, Noboru Matsuo, Yoshihisa Katsuragi, Masanori Komikado et al. "Green tea catechin consumption enhances exercise-induced abdominal fat loss in overweight and obese adults." The Journal of nutrition 139, no. 2 (2009): 264-270.

136. Zhu, B. T., J-Y. Shim, M. Nagai, and H-W. Bai. "Molecular modelling study of the mechanism of high-potency inhibition of human catechol-O-methyltransferase by (-)-epigallocatechin-3-O-gallate." Xenobiotica 38, no. 2 (2008): 130-146.

137. Phung, Olivia J., William L. Baker, Leslie J. Matthews, Michael Lanosa, Alicia Thorne, and Craig I. Coleman. "Effect of green tea catechins with or without caffeine on anthropometric measures: a systematic review and meta-analysis."The American journal of clinical nutrition 91, no. 1 (2010): 73-81.

138. Chow, HH Sherry, Iman A. Hakim, Donna R. Vining, James A. Crowell, James Ranger-Moore, Wade M. Chew, Catherine A. Celaya, Steven R. Rodney, Yukihiko Hara, and David S. Alberts. "Effects of dosing condition on the oral bioavailability of green tea catechins after single-dose administration of Polyphenon E in healthy individuals." Clinical Cancer Research 11, no. 12 (2005): 4627-4633.

139. Millan, Mark J., Adrian Newman-Tancredi, Valerie Audinot, Didier Cussac, Francoise Lejeune, Jean-Paul Nicolas, Francis Cogé et al. "Agonist and antagonist actions of yohimbine as compared to fluparoxan at α2-adrenergic receptors (AR) s, serotonin (5-HT) 1A, 5-HT1B, 5-HT1D and dopamine D2 and D3 receptors. Significance for the modulation of frontocortical monoaminergic transmission and depressive states." Synapse 35, no. 2 (2000): 79-95.

140. Ostojic, Sergej M. "Yohimbine: the effects on body composition and exercise performance in soccer players." Research in Sports Medicine 14, no. 4 (2006): 289-299.

141. Galitzky, J., M. Taouis, M. Berlan, D. Riviere, M. Garrigues, and M. Lafontan. "α2-

Antagonist compounds and lipid mobilization: evidence for a lipid mobilizing effect of oral yohimbine in healthy male volunteers." European journal of clinical investigation 18, no. 6 (1988): 587-594.

142. Ibid.

143. Galitzky, J., M. Taouis, M. Berlan, D. Riviere, M. Garrigues, and M. Lafontan. "α2-Antagonist compounds and lipid mobilization: evidence for a lipid mobilizing effect of oral yohimbine in healthy male volunteers." European journal of clinical investigation 18, no. 6 (1988): 587-594.

144. McCarty, Mark F. "Pre-exercise administration of yohimbine may enhance the efficacy of exercise training as a fat loss strategy by boosting lipolysis."Medical hypotheses 58, no. 6 (2002): 491-495.

145. Goldberg, MICHAEL R., ALAN S. Hollister, and D. A. V. I. D. Robertson. "Influence of yohimbine on blood pressure, autonomic reflexes, and plasma catecholamines in humans." Hypertension 5, no. 5 (1983): 772-778.

146. Haaz, S., K. R. Fontaine, G. Cutter, N. Limdi, S. Perumean-Chaney, and D. B. Allison. "Citrus aurantium and synephrine alkaloids in the treatment of overweight and obesity: an update." Obesity reviews 7, no. 1 (2006): 79-88.

147. Brown, C. M., J. C. McGrath, J. M. Midgley, A. G. B. Muir, J. W. O'Brien, C. M. Thonoor, C. M. Williams, and V. G. Wilson. "Activities of octopamine and synephrine stereoisomers on α-adrenoceptors." British journal of pharmacology93, no. 2 (1988): 417-429.

148. Gougeon, Réjeanne, Kathy Harrigan, Jean-François Tremblay, Philip Hedrei, Marie Lamarche, and José A. Morais. "Increase in the thermic effect of food in women by adrenergic amines extracted from citrus aurantium." Obesity research 13, no. 7 (2005): 1187-1194.

149. Seifert, John G., Aaron Nelson, Julia Devonish, Edmund R. Burke, and Sidney J. Stohs. "Effect of acute administration of an herbal preparation on blood pressure and heart rate in humans." International journal of medical sciences 8, no. 3 (2011): 192.

150. Williams, Jonathan, and Sohrab Mobarhan. "A critical interaction: leptin and ghrelin." Nutrition reviews 61, no. 11 (2003): 391-393.

151. Weigle, David S., David E. Cummings, Patricia D. Newby, Patricia A. Breen, R. Scott Frayo, Colleen C. Matthys, Holly S. Callahan, and Jonathan Q. Purnell. "Roles of leptin and ghrelin in the loss of body weight caused by a low fat, high carbohydrate diet." Journal of Clinical Endocrinology & Metabolism 88, no. 4 (2003): 1577-1586.

152. Jéquier, Eric. "Leptin signaling, adiposity, and energy balance." Annals of the New York Academy of Sciences 967, no. 1 (2002): 379-388.

153. Weigle, David S., Patricia A. Breen, Colleen C. Matthys, Holly S. Callahan, Kaatje E. Meeuws, Verna R. Burden, and Jonathan Q. Purnell. "A high-protein diet induces sustained reductions in appetite, ad libitum caloric intake, and body weight despite compensatory changes in diurnal plasma leptin and ghrelin concentrations." The American journal of clinical nutrition 82, no. 1 (2005): 41-48.

154. Dirlewanger, M., V. Di Vetta, E. Guenat, P. Battilana, G. Seematter, P. Schneiter, E. Jéquier, and L. Tappy. "Effects of short-term carbohydrate or fat overfeeding on energy expenditure and plasma leptin concentrations in healthy female subjects." International Journal of Obesity & Related Metabolic Disorders 24, no. 11 (2000).

155. Havel, Peter J., Raymond Townsend, Leslie Chaump, and Karen Teff. "High-fat meals

reduce 24-h circulating leptin concentrations in women." Diabetes 48, no. 2 (1999): 334-341.

156. Lin, L., R. Martin, A. O. Schaffhauser, and D. A. York. "Acute changes in the response to peripheral leptin with alteration in the diet composition." American Journal of Physiology-Regulatory, Integrative and Comparative Physiology 280, no. 2 (2001): R504-R509.

157. Dirlewanger, M., V. Di Vetta, E. Guenat, P. Battilana, G. Seematter, P. Schneiter, E. Jéquier, and L. Tappy. "Effects of short-term carbohydrate or fat overfeeding on energy expenditure and plasma leptin concentrations in healthy female subjects." International Journal of Obesity & Related Metabolic Disorders 24, no. 11 (2000).

158. Weigle, David S., David E. Cummings, Patricia D. Newby, Patricia A. Breen, R. Scott Frayo, Colleen C. Matthys, Holly S. Callahan, and Jonathan Q. Purnell. "Roles of leptin and ghrelin in the loss of body weight caused by a low fat, high carbohydrate diet." Journal of Clinical Endocrinology & Metabolism 88, no. 4 (2003): 1577-1586.

159. Astrup, Arne, Louise Ryan, Gary K. Grunwald, Mette Storgaard, Wim Saris, Ed Melanson, and James O. Hill. "The role of dietary fat in body fatness: evidence from a preliminary meta-analysis of ad libitum low-fat dietary intervention studies." British Journal of Nutrition 83, no. S1 (2000): S25-S32.

160. Burton-Freeman, Britt. "Dietary fiber and energy regulation." The Journal of nutrition 130, no. 2 (2000): 272S-275S.

161. Institute of Medicine (US). Panel on Macronutrients, and Institute of Medicine (US). Standing Committee on the Scientific Evaluation of Dietary Reference Intakes. Dietary reference intakes for energy, carbohydrate, fiber, fat, fatty acids, cholesterol, protein, and amino acids. Vol. 1. Natl Academy Pr, 2005.

162. Flores-Mateo, Gemma, David Rojas-Rueda, Josep Basora, Emilio Ros, and Jordi Salas-Salvadó. "Nut intake and adiposity: meta-analysis of clinical trials." The American journal of clinical nutrition 97, no. 6 (2013): 1346-1355.

163. Lappalainen, R., L. Mennen, L. Van Weert, and H. Mykkänen. "Drinking water with a meal: a simple method of coping with feelings of hunger, satiety and desire to eat." European journal of clinical nutrition 47, no. 11 (1993): 815-819.

164. Ludwig, David S., Joseph A. Majzoub, Ahmad Al-Zahrani, Gerard E. Dallal, Isaac Blanco, and Susan B. Roberts. "High glycemic index foods, overeating, and obesity." Pediatrics 103, no. 3 (1999): e26-e26.

165. Andrade, Ana M., Geoffrey W. Greene, and Kathleen J. Melanson. "Eating slowly led to decreases in energy intake within meals in healthy women." Journal of the American Dietetic Association 108, no. 7 (2008): 1186-1191.

166. Taheri, Shahrad, Ling Lin, Diane Austin, Terry Young, and Emmanuel Mignot. "Short sleep duration is associated with reduced leptin, elevated ghrelin, and increased body mass index." PLoS medicine 1, no. 3 (2004): e62.

167. Ibid.

168. A. G. Dulloo and L. Girardier. "Adaptive Changes in Energy Expenditure During Refeeding Following Low-Calorie Intake: Evidence for a Specific Metabolic Component Favoring Fat Storage," American Journal of Clinical Nutrition 52, no. 3 (1990): 415-420. http://ajcn.nutrition.org/content/52/3/415.short.

169. Stefan M. Pasiakos, Lisa M. Vislocky, John W. Carbone, Nicholas Altieri, Karen

Konopelski, Hedley C. Freake, Jeffrey M. Anderson, Arny A. Ferrando, Robert R. Wolfe, and Nancy R. Rodriguez. "Acute Energy Deprivation Affects Skeletal Muscle Protein Synthesis and Associated Intracellular Signaling Proteins in Physically Active Adults," Journal of Nutrition 140, no. 4 (2010): 745-751. doi:10.3945/jn.109.118372.

170. S. L. Miller and R. R. Wolfe. "Physical Exercise as a Modulator of Adaptation to Low and High Carbohydrate and Low and High Fat Intakes," European Journal of Clinical Nutrition 53 (1999): S112-S119.

171. A. Garg, A. Bonanome, S. M. Grundy, Z. J. Zhang, and R. H. Unger. "Comparison of a High-Carbohydrate Diet with a High-Monounsaturated-Fat Diet in Patients with Non-Insulin-Dependent Diabetes Mellitus," New England Journal of Medicine 319, no. 13 (1988): 829-834.

172. Joanne F. Dorgan, Joseph T. Judd, Christopher Longcope, Charles Brown, Arthur Schatzkin, Beverly A. Clevidence, William S. Campbell, Padmanabhan P. Nair, Charlene Franz, Lisa Kahle, and Philip R. Taylor. "Effects of Dietary Fat and Fiber on Plasma and Urine Androgens and Estrogens in Men: A Controlled Feeding Study," American Journal of Clinical Nutrition 64, no. 6 (1996): 850-855.

173. Robert A. Robergs, David R. Pearson, David L. Costill, William J. Fink, David D. Pascoe, Michael A. Benedict, Charles P. Lambert, and Jeffrey J. Zachweija. "Muscle Glycogenolysis During Differing Intensities of Weight-Resistance Exercise," Journal of Applied Physiology 70, no. 4 (1985): 1700-1706.

174. Ivy, J. L. "Glycogen resynthesis after exercise: effect of carbohydrate intake." International journal of sports medicine 19, no. 2 (1998): S142.

175. Ibid.

176. Wang, Xiaonan, Zhaoyong Hu, Junping Hu, Jie Du, and William E. Mitch. "Insulin resistance accelerates muscle protein degradation: Activation of the ubiquitin-proteasome pathway by defects in muscle cell signaling." Endocrinology 147, no. 9 (2006): 4160-4168.

177. Zhang, Jin, Christopher J. Hupfeld, Susan S. Taylor, Jerrold M. Olefsky, and Roger Y. Tsien. "Insulin disrupts β-adrenergic signalling to protein kinase A in adipocytes." Nature 437, no. 7058 (2005): 569-573.

178. Evans, William J., and Virginia A. Hughes. "Dietary carbohydrates and endurance exercise." The American journal of clinical nutrition 41, no. 5 (1985): 1146-1154.

179. Miller, S. L., and R. R. Wolfe. "Physical exercise as a modulator of adaptation to low and high carbohydrate and low and high fat intakes." European journal of clinical nutrition 53 (1999): S112-9.

180. Krista R. Howarth, Stuart M. Phillips, Maureen J. MacDonald, Douglas Richards, Natalie A. Moreau, and Martin J. Gibala. "Effect of Glycogen Availability on Human Skeletal Muscle Protein Turnover During Exercise and Recovery," Journal of Applied Physiology 109, no. 2 (2010): 431-438. doi: 10.1152/japplphysiol.00108.2009.

181. René Koopman, Milou Beelen, Trent Stellingwerff, Bart Pennings, Wim H. M. Saris, Arie K. Kies, Harm Kuipers, and Luc J. C. van Loon. "Coingestion of Carbohydrate with Protein Does Not Further Augment Postexercise Muscle Protein Synthesis," American Journal of Physiology—Endocrinology and Metabolism 293, no. E833-E842 (2007): E833-E842. doi: 10.1152/ajpendo.00135.2007.

182. Stuart M. Phillips. "Insulin and Muscle Protein Turnover in Humans: Stimulatory, Permissive, Inhibitory, or All of the Above?" American Journal of Physiology—

Endocrinology and Metabolism 295, no. E731 (2008). doi: 10.1152/ajpendo.90569.2008.

183. Krista R. Howarth, Stuart M. Phillips, Maureen J. MacDonald, Douglas Richards, Natalie A. Moreau, and Martin J. Gibala. "Effect of Glycogen Availability on Human Skeletal Muscle Protein Turnover During Exercise and Recovery," Journal of Applied Physiology 109, no. 2 (2010): 431-438. doi: 10.1152/japplphysiol.00108.2009.

184. Michelle N. Harvie, Mary Pegington, Mark P. Mattson, Jan Frystyk, Bernice Dillon, Gareth Evans, Jack Cuzick, Susan A. Jebb, Bronwen Martin, Roy G. Cutler, Tae G. Son, Stuart Maudsley, Olga D. Carlson, Josephine M. Egan, Allan Flyvbjerg, and Anthony Howell. "The Effects of Intermittent or Continuous Energy Restriction on Weight Loss and Metabolic Disease Risk Markers: A Randomised Trial in Young Overweight Women," International Journal of Obesity 35, no. 5 (2011): 714-727. doi: 10.1038/ijo.2010.171.

185. Sudesh Kumar Yadav and Praveen Guleria. "Steviol Glycosides from Stevia: Biosynthesis Pathway Review and Their Application in Foods and Medicine," Critical Reviews in Food Science and Nutrition 52, no. 11 (2012): 988-998. doi: 10.1080/10408398.2010.519447.

186. Richard A. Anderson. "Chromium and Polyphenols from Cinnamon Improve Insulin Sensitivity," Proceedings of the Nutrition Society 67, no. 1 (1985): 48-53. doi: 10.1017/S0029665108006010.

187. José C. E. Serrano, Hugo Gonzalo-Benito, Mariona Jové, Stéphane Fourcade, Anna Cassanyé, Jordi Boada, Marco A. Delgado, Alberto E. Espinel, Reinald Pamplona, and Manuel Portero-Otín. "Dietary intake of Green Tea Polyphenols Regulates Insulin Sensitivity with an Increase in AMP-Activated Protein Kinase α Content and Changes in Mitochondrial Respiratory Complexes," Molecular Nutrition and Food Research 57, no. 3 (2013): 459-470. doi: 10.1002/mnfr.201200513.

188. Tao Huang, Mark L. Wahlqvist, Tongcheng Xu, Amei Xu, Aizhen Zhang, and Duo Li. "Increased Plasma n-3 Polyunsaturated Fatty Acid Is Associated with Improved Insulin Sensitivity in Type 2 Diabetes in China," Molecular Nutrition and Food Research 54, no. 1 (2010): S112-S119. doi: 10.1002/mnfr.200900189.

189. Azabji-Kenfack Marcel, Loni G. Ekali, Sobngwi Eugene, Onana E. Arnold, Edie D. Sandrine, Denis Von der Weid, Emmanuel Gbaguidi, Jeanne Ngogang, and Jean C. Mbanya. "The Effect of Spirulina platensis versus Soybean on Insulin Resistance in HIV-Infected Patients: A Randomized Pilot Study," Nutrients 3, no. 7 (2011): 712-724. doi: 10.3390/nu3070712.

190. Siri-Tarino, Patty W., Qi Sun, Frank B. Hu, and Ronald M. Krauss. "Meta-analysis of prospective cohort studies evaluating the association of saturated fat with cardiovascular disease." The American journal of clinical nutrition 91, no. 3 (2010): 535-546.

191. Margriet S. Westerterp-Plantenga. "The Significance of Protein in Food Intake and Body Weight Regulation," Current Opinion in Clinical Nutrition & Metabolic Care 6, no. 6 (2003): 635-638.

192. Poortmans, Jacques R., and Olivier Dellalieux. "Do regular high protein diets have potential health risks on kidney function in athletes?." International Journal of Sport Nutrition 10, no. 1 (2000): 28-38.

193. Soeters, Maarten R., Nicolette M. Lammers, Peter F. Dubbelhuis, Mariëtte Ackermans, Cora F. Jonkers-Schuitema, Eric Fliers, Hans P. Sauerwein, Johannes M. Aerts, and Mireille J. Serlie. "Intermittent fasting does not affect whole-body glucose, lipid, or protein metabolism." The American journal of clinical nutrition 90, no. 5 (2009): 1244-1251.

194. http://www.acnp.org/g4/gn401000064/ch064.html

195. Cahill Jr, Geprge F. "Starvation in man." The New England journal of medicine 282, no. 12 (1970): 668-

196. Bilsborough, Shane, and Neil Mann. "A review of issues of dietary protein intake in humans." International journal of sport nutrition and exercise metabolism 16, no. 2 (2006): 129.

197. Nair, K. S., P. D. Woolf, S. L. Welle, and D. E. Matthews. "Leucine, glucose, and energy metabolism after 3 days of fasting in healthy human subjects." The American journal of clinical nutrition 46, no. 4 (1987): 557-562.

198. Zauner, Christian, Bruno Schneeweiss, Alexander Kranz, Christian Madl, Klaus Ratheiser, Ludwig Kramer, Erich Roth, Barbara Schneider, and Kurt Lenz. "Resting energy expenditure in short-term starvation is increased as a result of an increase in serum norepinephrine." The American journal of clinical nutrition 71, no. 6 (2000): 1511-1515.

199. Owen, Oliver E., Karl J. Smalley, David A. D'Alessio, Maria A. Mozzoli, and Elizabeth K. Dawson. "Protein, fat, and carbohydrate requirements during starvation: anaplerosis and cataplerosis." The American journal of clinical nutrition 68, no. 1 (1998): 12-34.

200. Varady, Krista A., and Marc K. Hellerstein. "Alternate-day fasting and chronic disease prevention: a review of human and animal trials." The American journal of clinical nutrition 86, no. 1 (2007): 7-13.

201. Harvie, Michelle N., Mary Pegington, Mark P. Mattson, Jan Frystyk, Bernice Dillon, Gareth Evans, Jack Cuzick et al. "The effects of intermittent or continuous energy restriction on weight loss and metabolic disease risk markers: a randomized trial in young overweight women." International journal of obesity 35, no. 5 (2011): 714-727.

202. Hartman, MARK L., JOHANNES D. Veldhuis, MICHAEL L. Johnson, MARY M. Lee, K. G. Alberti, E. U. G. E. N. E. Samojlik, and M. O. Thorner. "Augmented growth hormone (GH) secretory burst frequency and amplitude mediate enhanced GH secretion during a two-day fast in normal men." The Journal of clinical endocrinology and metabolism 74, no. 4 (1992): 757-765.

203. Derave, Wim, Ann Mertens, Erik Muls, Karel Pardaens, and Peter Hespel. "Effects of Post-absorptive and Postprandial Exercise on Glucoregulation in Metabolic Syndrome." Obesity 15, no. 3 (2007): 704-711.

204. Mattson, Mark P., Wenzhen Duan, and Zhihong Guo. "Meal size and frequency affect neuronal plasticity and vulnerability to disease: cellular and molecular mechanisms." Journal of neurochemistry 84, no. 3 (2003): 417-431.

205. Aksungar, Fehime B., Aynur E. Topkaya, and Mahmut Akyildiz. "Interleukin-6, C-reactive protein and biochemical parameters during prolonged intermittent fasting." Annals of Nutrition and Metabolism 51, no. 1 (2007): 88-95.

206. Masiero, Eva, Lisa Agatea, Cristina Mammucari, Bert Blaauw, Emanuele Loro, Masaaki Komatsu, Daniel Metzger, Carlo Reggiani, Stefano Schiaffino, and Marco Sandri. "Autophagy is required to maintain muscle mass." Cell metabolism 10, no. 6 (2009): 507-515.

207. Bergamini, Ettore, Gabriella Cavallini, Alessio Donati, and Zina Gori. "The role of autophagy in aging." Annals of the New York Academy of Sciences 1114, no. 1 (2007): 69-78.

208. Stote, Kim S., David J. Baer, Karen Spears, David R. Paul, G. Keith Harris, William V. Rumpler, Pilar Strycula et al. "A controlled trial of reduced meal frequency without caloric restriction in healthy, normal-weight, middle-aged adults." The American journal of clinical nutrition 85, no. 4 (2007): 981-988.

209. Ibid.

210. Faintuch, Joel, Francisco Garcia Soriano, José Paulo Ladeira, Mariano Janiszewski, Irineu Tadeu Velasco, and Joaquim J. Gama-Rodrigues. "Changes in body fluid and energy compartments during prolonged hunger strike." Revista do Hospital das Clínicas 55, no. 2 (2000): 47-54.

211. Carroll, Sean, and Mike Dudfield. "What is the Relationship Between Exercise and Metabolic Abnormalities?." Sports Medicine 34, no. 6 (2004): 371-418.

212. http://www.leangains.com/2010/04/leangains-guide.html

213. Chow, Lisa S., Robert C. Albright, Maureen L. Bigelow, Gianna Toffolo, Claudio Cobelli, and K. Sreekumaran Nair. "Mechanism of insulin's anabolic effect on muscle: measurements of muscle protein synthesis and breakdown using aminoacyl-tRNA and other surrogate measures." American Journal of Physiology-Endocrinology and Metabolism 291, no. 4 (2006): E729-E736.

214. Ibid.

215. Sacks, Frank M., George A. Bray, Vincent J. Carey, Steven R. Smith, Donna H. Ryan, Stephen D. Anton, Katherine McManus et al. "Comparison of weight-loss diets with different compositions of fat, protein, and carbohydrates." New England Journal of Medicine 360, no. 9 (2009): 859-873.

216. Johnston, Carol S., Sherrie L. Tjonn, Pamela D. Swan, Andrea White, Heather Hutchins, and Barry Sears. "Ketogenic low-carbohydrate diets have no metabolic advantage over nonketogenic low-carbohydrate diets." The American journal of clinical nutrition 83, no. 5 (2006): 1055-1061.

217. Mason, Caitlin, Karen E. Foster-Schubert, Ikuyo Imayama, Angela Kong, Liren Xiao, Carolyn Bain, Kristin L. Campbell et al. "Dietary weight loss and exercise effects on insulin resistance in postmenopausal women." American journal of preventive medicine 41, no. 4 (2011): 366-375.

218. Chow, Lisa S., Robert C. Albright, Maureen L. Bigelow, Gianna Toffolo, Claudio Cobelli, and K. Sreekumaran Nair. "Mechanism of insulin's anabolic effect on muscle: measurements of muscle protein synthesis and breakdown using aminoacyl-tRNA and other surrogate measures." American Journal of Physiology-Endocrinology and Metabolism 291, no. 4 (2006): E729-E736.

219. Katzeff, Harvey L., Maureen O'Connell, Edward S. Horton, Elliot Danforth Jr, James B. Young, and Lewis Landsberg. "Metabolic studies in human obesity during overnutrition and undernutrition: thermogenic and hormonal responses to norepinephrine." Metabolism 35, no. 2 (1986): 166-175.

220. Keller, Andreas, Angela Graefen, Markus Ball, Mark Matzas, Valesca Boisguerin, Frank Maixner, Petra Leidinger et al. "New insights into the Tyrolean Iceman's origin and phenotype as inferred by whole-genome sequencing." Nature communications 3 (2012): 698.

221. http://news.nationalgeographic.com/news/2010/08/100831-cannibalism-cannibal-cavemen-human-meat-science/

222. Cordain, Loren, Janette Brand Miller, S. Boyd Eaton, Neil Mann, Susanne HA Holt, and John D. Speth. "Plant-animal subsistence ratios and macronutrient energy estimations in worldwide hunter-gatherer diets." The American journal of clinical nutrition 71, no. 3 (2000): 682-692.

223. Murdock, George Peter. "Ethnographic atlas: A summary." Ethnology (1967): 109-236.

224. Milton, Katharine. "Hunter-gatherer diets—a different perspective." The American journal of clinical nutrition 71, no. 3 (2000): 665-667.

225. Henry, Amanda G., Peter S. Ungar, Benjamin H. Passey, Matt Sponheimer, Lloyd Rossouw, Marion Bamford, Paul Sandberg, Darryl J. de Ruiter, and Lee Berger. "The diet of Australopithecus sediba." Nature (2012).

226. Mercader, Julio. "Mozambican grass seed consumption during the Middle Stone Age." Science 326, no. 5960 (2009): 1680-1683.

227. Henry, Amanda G., Alison S. Brooks, and Dolores R. Piperno. "Microfossils in calculus demonstrate consumption of plants and cooked foods in Neanderthal diets (Shanidar III, Iraq; Spy I and II, Belgium)." Proceedings of the National Academy of Sciences 108, no. 2 (2011): 486-491.

228. Revedin, Anna, Biancamaria Aranguren, Roberto Becattini, Laura Longo, Emanuele Marconi, Marta Mariotti Lippi, Natalia Skakun, Andrey Sinitsyn, Elena Spiridonova, and Jiří Svoboda. "Thirty thousand-year-old evidence of plant food processing." Proceedings of the National Academy of Sciences 107, no. 44 (2010): 18815-18819.

229. http://thepaleodiet.com/paleo-diet-faq/

230. Volk, Marion G. "An examination of the evidence supporting the association of dietary cholesterol and saturated fats with serum cholesterol and development of coronary heart disease." Alternative Medicine Review 12, no. 3 (2007).

231. Westerterp-Plantenga, Margriet S. "The significance of protein in food intake and body weight regulation." Current Opinion in Clinical Nutrition & Metabolic Care 6, no. 6 (2003): 635-638.

232. Rohrmann, Sabine, Kim Overvad, H. Bas Bueno-de-Mesquita, Marianne U. Jakobsen, Rikke Egeberg, Anne Tjønneland, Laura Nailler et al. "Meat consumption and mortality-results from the European Prospective Investigation into Cancer and Nutrition." BMC medicine 11, no. 1 (2013): 63.

233. He, F. J., C. A. Nowson, M. Lucas, and G. A. MacGregor. "Increased consumption of fruit and vegetables is related to a reduced risk of coronary heart disease: meta-analysis of cohort studies." Journal of human hypertension21, no. 9 (2007): 717-728.

234. He, Feng J., Caryl A. Nowson, and Graham A. MacGregor. "Fruit and vegetable consumption and stroke: meta-analysis of cohort studies." The Lancet 367, no. 9507 (2006): 320-326.

235. Hamer, Mark, and Yoichi Chida. "Intake of fruit, vegetables, and antioxidants and risk of type 2 diabetes: systematic review and meta-analysis." Journal of hypertension 25, no. 12 (2007): 2361-2369.

236. Ramel, Alfons, J. Alfredo Martinez, Mairead Kiely, Narcisa M. Bandarra, and Inga Thorsdottir. "Moderate consumption of fatty fish reduces diastolic blood pressure in overweight and obese European young adults during energy restriction." Nutrition 26, no. 2 (2010): 168-174.

237. Muldoon, Matthew F., Christopher M. Ryan, Lei Sheu, Jeffrey K. Yao, Sarah M. Conklin, and Stephen B. Manuck. "Serum phospholipid docosahexaenonic acid is associated with cognitive functioning during middle adulthood." The Journal of nutrition 140, no. 4 (2010): 848-853.

238. Lauretani, F., M. Maggio, F. Pizzarelli, S. Michelassi, C. Ruggiero, G. P. Ceda, S. Bandinelli, and L. Ferrucci. "Omega-3 and renal function in older adults."Current pharmaceutical design 15, no. 36 (2009): 4149.

239. Simopoulos, Artemis P. "The importance of the omega-6/omega-3 fatty acid ratio in cardiovascular disease and other chronic diseases." Experimental Biology and Medicine 233, no. 6 (2008): 674-688.

240. He, Ka, Eric B. Rimm, Anwar Merchant, Bernard A. Rosner, Meir J. Stampfer, Walter C. Willett, and Alberto Ascherio. "Fish consumption and risk of stroke in men." Jama 288, no. 24 (2002): 3130-3136.

241. Huang, Tao, Subhachai Bhulaidok, Zhenzhen Cai, Tongcheng Xu, Fang Xu, Mark L. Wahlqvist, and Duo Li. "Plasma phospholipids n-3 polyunsaturated fatty acid is associated with metabolic syndrome." Molecular nutrition & food research 54, no. 11 (2010): 1628-1635.

242. Gibson, Sigrid A. "Dietary sugars intake and micronutrient adequacy: a systematic review of the evidence." Nutrition research reviews 20, no. 02 (2007): 121-131.

243. Barclay, Alan W., Peter Petocz, Joanna McMillan-Price, Victoria M. Flood, Tania Prvan, Paul Mitchell, and Jennie C. Brand-Miller. "Glycemic index, glycemic load, and chronic disease risk—a meta-analysis of observational studies." The American Journal of Clinical Nutrition 87, no. 3 (2008): 627-637.

244. Micha, R., and D. Mozaffarian. "Trans fatty acids: effects on cardiometabolic health and implications for policy." Prostaglandins, Leukotrienes and Essential Fatty Acids 79, no. 3 (2008): 147-152.

245. Frassetto, Lynda A., M. Schloetter, M. Mietus-Synder, R. C. Morris, and A. Sebastian. "Metabolic and physiologic improvements from consuming a paleolithic, hunter-gatherer type diet." European journal of clinical nutrition 63, no. 8 (2009): 947-955.

246. Lindeberg, Staffan, Tommy Jönsson, Yvonne Granfeldt, E. Borgstrand, J. Soffman, Kerstin Sjöström, and Bo Ahrén. "A Palaeolithic diet improves glucose tolerance more than a Mediterranean-like diet in individuals with ischaemic heart disease." Diabetologia 50, no. 9 (2007): 1795-1807.

247. Appel, Lawrence J. "Dietary Patterns and Longevity Expanding the Blue Zones."Circulation 118, no. 3 (2008): 214-215.

248. Heaney, Robert P. "Dairy and bone health." Journal of the American College of Nutrition 28, no. sup1 (2009): 82S-90S.

249. Josse, Andrea R., Jason E. Tang, Mark A. Tarnopolsky, and Stuart M. Phillips. "Body composition and strength changes in women with milk and resistance exercise." Med Sci Sports Exerc 42, no. 6 (2010): 1122-30.

250. Van Loan, Marta. "The role of dairy foods and dietary calcium in weight management." Journal of the American College of Nutrition 28, no. sup1 (2009): 120S-129S.

251. http://nutritionfacts.org/2011/09/08/how-much-pus-is-there-in-milk/

252. http://www.cancer.org/cancer/cancercauses/othercarcinogens/athome/recombinant-bovine-growth-hormone

253. Masters, Rachel C., Angela D. Liese, Steven M. Haffner, Lynne E. Wagenknecht, and Anthony J. Hanley. "Whole and refined grain intakes are related to inflammatory protein concentrations in human plasma." The Journal of nutrition 140, no. 3 (2010): 587-594.

254. Katcher, Heather I., Richard S. Legro, Allen R. Kunselman, Peter J. Gillies, Laurence M. Demers, Deborah M. Bagshaw, and Penny M. Kris-Etherton. "The effects of a whole grain–enriched hypocaloric diet on cardiovascular disease risk factors in men and women with metabolic syndrome." The American journal of clinical nutrition 87, no. 1 (2008): 79-90.

255. de Munter, Jeroen SL, Frank B. Hu, Donna Spiegelman, Mary Franz, and Rob M. van Dam. "Whole grain, bran, and germ intake and risk of type 2 diabetes: a prospective cohort study and systematic review." PLoS medicine 4, no. 8 (2007): e261.

256. Jacobs Jr, David R., Leonard Marquart, Joanne Slavin, and Lawrence H. Kushi. "Whole-grain intake and cancer: An expanded review and meta-analysis."Nutrition and cancer 30, no. 2 (1998): 85-96.

257. http://www.health.harvard.edu/newsweek/The_nutrients_that_are_lost_when_grain_is_refined.htm

258. Masters, Rachel C., Angela D. Liese, Steven M. Haffner, Lynne E. Wagenknecht, and Anthony J. Hanley. "Whole and refined grain intakes are related to inflammatory protein concentrations in human plasma." The Journal of nutrition 140, no. 3 (2010): 587-594.

259. Bazzano, Lydia A., Angela M. Thompson, Michael T. Tees, Cuong H. Nguyen, and Donna M. Winham. "Non-soy legume consumption lowers cholesterol levels: a meta-analysis of randomized controlled trials." Nutrition, Metabolism and Cardiovascular Diseases 21, no. 2 (2011): 94-103.

260. Gilani, G. Sarwar, Kevin A. Cockell, and Estatira Sepehr. "Effects of antinutritional factors on protein digestibility and amino acid availability in foods." Journal of AOAC International 88, no. 3 (2005): 967-987.

261. Hotz, Christine, and Rosalind S. Gibson. "Traditional food-processing and preparation practices to enhance the bioavailability of micronutrients in plant-based diets." The Journal of nutrition 137, no. 4 (2007): 1097-1100.

262. Gollnick, P. D., Karin Piehl, and B. Saltin. "Selective glycogen depletion pattern in human muscle fibres after exercise of varying intensity and at varying pedalling rates." The Journal of physiology 241, no. 1 (1974): 45-57.

263. Ivy, John L. "Regulation of muscle glycogen repletion, muscle protein synthesis and repair following exercise." Journal of Sports Science & Medicine 3, no. 3 (2004): 131.

264. Ivy, J. L. "Glycogen resynthesis after exercise: effect of carbohydrate intake."International journal of sports medicine 19, no. 2 (1998): S142.

265. Abou-Donia, Mohamed B., Eman M. El-Masry, Ali A. Abdel-Rahman, Roger E. McLendon, and Susan S. Schiffman. "Splenda alters gut microflora and increases intestinal p-glycoprotein and cytochrome p-450 in male rats." Journal of Toxicology and Environmental Health, Part A 71, no. 21 (2008): 1415-1429.

266. Qin, Xiaofa. "What made Canada become a country with the highest incidence of inflammatory bowel disease: Could sucralose be the culprit?." Canadian Journal of Gastroenterology 25, no. 9 (2011): 511.

267. Schernhammer, Eva S., Kimberly A. Bertrand, Brenda M. Birmann, Laura Sampson, Walter C. Willett, and Diane Feskanich. "Consumption of artificial sweetener–and sugar-containing soda and risk of lymphoma and leukemia in men and women." The American journal of clinical nutrition 96, no. 6 (2012): 1419-1428.

268. Fowler, Sharon P., Ken Williams, Roy G. Resendez, Kelly J. Hunt, Helen P. Hazuda, and Michael P. Stern. "Fueling the Obesity Epidemic? Artificially Sweetened Beverage Use and Long-term Weight Gain." Obesity 16, no. 8 (2008): 1894-1900.

269. Yadav, Sudesh Kumar, and Praveen Guleria. "Steviol glycosides from Stevia: biosynthesis pathway review and their application in foods and medicine."Critical reviews in food science and nutrition 52, no. 11 (2012): 988-998.

270. Shivanna, Naveen, Mahadev Naika, Farhath Khanum, and Vijay K. Kaul. "Antioxidant, anti-diabetic and renal protective properties of< i> Stevia rebaudiana</i>." Journal of Diabetes and its Complications 27, no. 2 (2013): 103-113.

271. FOOD, WHO. "Safety evaluation of certain food additives." (2010).

272. Ozbayer, Cansu, Hulyam Kurt, Suna Kalender, Hilmi Ozden, Hasan V. Gunes, Ayse Basaran, Ecir A. Cakmak, Kismet Civi, Yusuf Kalender, and Irfan Degirmenci. "Effects of Stevia rebaudiana (Bertoni) extract and N-nitro-L-arginine on renal function and ultrastructure of kidney cells in experimental type 2 Diabetes." Journal of medicinal food 14, no. 10 (2011): 1215-1222.

273. Feng, J., C. E. Cerniglia, and H. Chen. "Toxicological significance of azo dye metabolism by human intestinal microbiota." Frontiers in bioscience (Elite edition) 4 (2011): 568-586.

274. Tanaka, Toyohito, Osamu Takahashi, Shinshi Oishi, and Akio Ogata. "Effects of tartrazine on exploratory behavior in a three-generation toxicity study in mice." Reproductive Toxicology 26, no. 2 (2008): 156-163.

275. Kanarek, Robin B. "Artificial food dyes and attention deficit hyperactivity disorder." Nutrition reviews 69, no. 7 (2011): 385-391.

276. Moutinho, I. L. D., L. C. Bertges, and R. V. C. Assis. "Prolonged use of the food dye tartrazine (FD&C yellow n° 5) and its effects on the gastric mucosa of Wistar rats." Brazilian journal of biology 67, no. 1 (2007): 141-145.

277. Nigg, Joel T., Kara Lewis, Tracy Edinger, and Michael Falk. "Meta-analysis of attention-deficit/hyperactivity disorder or attention-deficit/hyperactivity disorder symptoms, restriction diet, and synthetic food color additives." Journal of the American Academy of Child & Adolescent Psychiatry 51, no. 1 (2012): 86-97.

66493414R00166

Made in the USA
Middletown, DE
12 March 2018